ONE STOP D Library

Statistics a

Epidemiolo

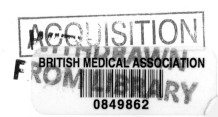

One Stop Doc

Titles in the series include:

Cardiovascular System – Jonathan Aron
Editorial Advisor – Jeremy Ward

Cell and Molecular Biology – Desikan Rangarajan and David Shaw
Editorial Advisor – Barbara Moreland

Endocrine and Reproductive Systems – Caroline Jewels and Alexandra Tillett
Editorial Advisor – Stuart Milligan

Gastrointestinal System – Miruna Canagaratnam
Editorial Advisor – Richard Naftalin

Musculoskeletal System – Wayne Lam, Bassel Zebian and Rishi Aggarwal
Editorial Advisor – Alistair Hunter

Nervous System – Elliott Smock
Editorial Advisor – Clive Coen

Metabolism and Nutrition – Miruna Canagaratnam and David Shaw
Editorial Advisors – Barbara Moreland and Richard Naftalin

Respiratory System – Jo Dartnell and Michelle Ramsay
Editorial Advisor – John Rees

Renal and Urinary System and Electrolyte Balance – Panos Stamoulos and Spyridon Bakalis
Editorial Advisors – Alistair Hunter and Richard Naftalin

Gastroenterology and Renal Medicine – Reena Popat and Danielle Adebayo
Editorial Advisor – Steve Pereira

Coming soon:

Cardiology – Rishi Aggarwal, Nina Muirhead and Emily Ferenczi
Editorial Advisor – Darrell Francis

Respiratory Medicine – Rameen Shakur and Ashraf Khan
Editorial Advisors – Nikhil Hirani and John Simpson

Immunology – Stephen Boag and Amy Sadler
Editorial Advisor – John Stewart

ONE STOP DOC

Statistics and Epidemiology

Emily Ferenczi BA(Cantab)
Sixth Year Medical Student, Oxford University Clinical School, Oxford, UK

Nina Muirhead BA(Oxon)
Sixth Year Medical Student, Oxford University Clinical School, Oxford, UK

Editorial Advisor: Lucy Carpenter BA MSc PhD
Reader in Statistical Epidemiology, Department of Public Health, Oxford University, Oxford, UK

Series Editor: Elliott Smock MB BS BSc(Hons)
House Officer (FY1), Eastbourne District General Hospital, Eastbourne, UK

Hodder Arnold

A MEMBER OF THE HODDER HEADLINE GROUP

First published in Great Britain in 2006 by
Hodder Arnold, an imprint of Hodder Education and a member of the Hodder Headline Group,
338 Euston Road, London NW1 3BH

http://www.hoddereducation.com

Distributed in the United States of America by
Oxford University Press Inc.,
198 Madison Avenue, New York, NY10016
Oxford is a registered trademark of Oxford University Press

Whilst the advice and information in this book are believed to be true and
accurate at the date of going to press, neither the author[s] nor the publisher
can accept any legal responsibility or liability for any errors or omissions
that may be made. In particular, (but without limiting the generality of the
preceding disclaimer) every effort has been made to check drug dosages;
however it is still possible that errors have been missed. Furthermore,
dosage schedules are constantly being revised and new side-effects
recognized. For these reasons the reader is strongly urged to consult the
drug companies' printed instructions before administering any of the drugs
recommended in this book.

British Library Cataloguing in Publication Data
A catalogue record for this book is available from the British Library

Library of Congress Cataloging-in-Publication Data
A catalog record for this book is available from the Library of Congress

ISBN-10 0340 92554 X
ISBN-13 978 0340 92554 6

1 2 3 4 5 6 7 8 9 10

Commissioning Editor: Christina De Bono
Project Editor: Clare Weber, Jane Tod
Production Controller: Lindsay Smith
Cover Design: Amina Dudhia
Indexer: Jane Gilbert, Indexing Specialists (UK) Ltd

Typeset in 10/12pt Adobe Garamond/Akzidenz GroteskBE by Servis Filmsetting Ltd, Manchester
Printed and bound in Spain

Hodder Headline's policy is to use papers that are natural, renewable and recyclable
products and made from wood grown in sustainable forests. The logging and manufacturing processes are
expected to conform to the environmental regulations of the country of origin.

What do you think about this book? Or any other Hodder Arnold title?
Please visit our website at **www.hoddereducation.com**

CONTENTS

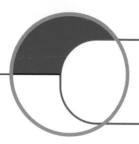

PREFACE

From the Series Editor, Elliott Smock

Are you ready to face your looming exams? If you have done loads of work, then congratulations; we hope this opportunity to practise SAQs, EMQs, MCQs and Problem-based Questions on every part of the core curriculum will help you consolidate what you've learnt and improve your exam technique. If you don't feel ready, don't panic – the One Stop Doc series has all the answers you need to catch up and pass.

There are only a limited number of questions an examiner can throw at a beleaguered student and this text can turn that to your advantage. By getting straight into the heart of the core questions that come up year after year and by giving you the model answers you need, this book will arm you with the knowledge to succeed in your exams. Broken down into logical sections, you can learn all the important facts you need to pass without having to wade through tons of different textbooks when you simply don't have the time. All questions presented here are 'core'; those of the highest importance have been highlighted to allow even sharper focus if time for revision is running out. In addition, to allow you to organize your revision efficiently, questions have been grouped by topic, with answers supported by detailed integrated explanations.

On behalf of all the One Stop Doc authors I wish you the very best of luck in your exams and hope these books serve you well!

From the Authors, Emily Ferenczi and Nina Muirhead

In our first year of medical school, we remember groaning at the thought of having a statistics lecture. It all seemed so irrelevant and abstract at the time. However, after several years of essays, critical reviews and projects, we have come to appreciate the value of statistics. So much so in fact, that we were inspired to write a book about it! In the hospital, hearing doctors talk to patients about the evidence they have for offering one particular treatment over another, we realised that 'evidence-based medicine' is not just a fantasy, but a real and important aspect of the way we should approach medical practice throughout our careers.

In this book, we have used examples from recent medical literature to provide both inspiration and practical examples of the way statistics and epidemiological methods are used in clinical studies to guide clinical practice. The aim of this book is to equip medical students with an understanding and a tool guide for reading and reviewing clinical studies so that, as practising doctors, they can arrive at valid conclusions and make justifiable clinical decisions based upon the available evidence. It also aims to provide a basis by which a medical student or junior doctor can learn about starting a clinical study and how to access the information and resources that they need.

We have chosen published studies to illustrate important epidemiological and statistical concepts. Please bear in mind that the studies are chosen on the basis of their ability to demonstrate key issues that arise when analysing different study designs, not necessarily on the basis of their quality.

We would like to thank Adrian Smith for his very helpful comments on the draft document.

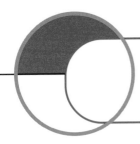

ABBREVIATIONS

ANOVA	analysis of variance
BMI	body mass index
CFTR	cystic fibrosis transmembrane conductance regulator
CI	confidence interval
df	degrees of freedom
FEV_1	forced expiratory volume
FN	false negative
FP	false positive
F/T PSA	free-to-total prostate-specific antigen
GP	general practitioner
H_0	null hypothesis
H_1	alternative hypothesis
HbA_{1c}	haemoglobin A_{1c}
HIV	human immunodeficiency virus
MHRA	Medicines and Healthcare products Regulatory Agency
MI	myocardial infarction
MMR	measles, mumps and rubella
NHS	National Health Service
NNT	numbers needed to treat
NPV	negative predictive value
OR	odds ratio
PPV	positive predictive value
PSA	prostate-specific antigen
RSI	repetitive strain injury
SD	standard deviation
SE	standard error
SEM	standard error of the mean
SE(p)	standard error of the proportion
SSRI	selective serotonin reuptake inhibitor
TN	true negative
TP	true positive

PART 1

EPIDEMIOLOGY

1

STUDYING HEALTH AND DISEASE IN POPULATIONS

STUDYING HEALTH AND DISEASE IN POPULATIONS

1. What is the definition of epidemiology and what are its uses?

2. What is meant by the following terms and how do they differ from each other?

    a. The distribution of disease   **b.** The determinants of disease

3. Which type of information would provide you with an idea of the distribution of the disease in developing versus developed countries?

    a. A case–control study
    b. A randomized controlled trial
    c. The National Infant Mortality Register
    d. The National Cancer Register
    e. An ecological study into the correlation between infectious disease rate and population density

4. Which type of information would help you to understand the determinants of breast cancer?

    a. A case–control study investigating the correlation between use of hormonal contraception and the risk of breast cancer
    b. The National Cancer Register
    c. A cohort study into the incidence of breast cancer in two groups of women: in one group, all the women have a family history of breast cancer, in the second group, there is no family history
    d. An ecological study comparing the rates of breast cancer in the UK and in France
    e. A randomized controlled trial investigating the efficacy of a new drug treatment for breast cancer

5. Identify the numerators and denominators in the following scenarios

    a. In a school of 670 children, 380 eat lunch in the canteen, 8 children have been identified as having gastroenteritis as a result of one of the canteen's chicken dishes
    b. A country has a population of 20 million people. Of these, 10 million live in highly polluted cities. 450 000 have been diagnosed with pollution-induced asthma
    c. A study wants to investigate the association between smoking and infertility using data on couples. There are 340 couples enrolled in a fertility clinic; 120 couples are defined as smokers (one or both partners smoke)

EXPLANATION: PRINCIPLES OF EPIDEMIOLOGY

Epidemiology is the quantitative study of the distribution and determinants of health and disease in a population **(1)**.

Analytic epidemiological studies typically involve four components: the definition of disease and identification of the 'at risk' population; the measurement of disease; the measurement of exposure and the examination of the association between disease and exposure.

Understanding of the distribution and determinants of health problems in populations can help direct public health strategies, for the prevention and treatment of disease, to improve the health of a population. It can ensure that money is spent in the right way on the people who are at risk **(1)**.

Any epidemiological parameter requires two numbers: a **numerator**, such as the number of individuals who have been defined as having a disease and a **denominator**, the defined population from which these individuals have been taken. Information on both the numerator and the denominator is crucial in epidemiology.

To illustrate: '10 people have been diagnosed with skin cancer in one month' – this figure is meaningless if one does not know from what size population these 10 people have been identified. A population of only 20 individuals may raise more concern than a population of 20 million individuals.

Different populations and subgroups of populations are affected by different health problems to different extents. Information about the **distribution of health problems** can be obtained through routinely collected data such as censuses and registers for death and disease, and through cross-sectional prevalence surveys **(2a)**.

Establishing the **determinants of health and disease** is based upon identifying the association between an individual's exposure to specific risk or protective factors and the subsequent health outcome for that individual **(2b)**. Ecological studies investigate exposure and disease at the level of population groups, rather than at the level of the individual. Studies that record exposure and disease status of individuals within a population include:
• Cross-sectional studies, which measure disease exposure
• Case–control studies
• Cohort studies.

Epidemiological evidence provides an idea of the extent and burden of health problems in a population, and thus can be used to direct public health strategies and treatment programmes aimed at improving health and reducing disease. Studies that investigate the effects of an intervention on health status include randomized controlled clinical trials of individual communities.

Answers

1. See explanation
2. See explanation
3. F F T T T
4. T F T T F

5. a – Numerator: 8 cases, denominator: 380 children at risk from canteen food, b – Numerator: 450 000 cases, denominator: 10 million in 'at risk' population, c – Numerator: 120 couples who are smokers (cases), denominator: 340 infertile couples (population of interest)

6. Define prevalence and incidence

7. Calculate the prevalence of

 a. Smoking in medical students: sample of 170 medical students, 38 smokers, 132 non-smokers
 b. Repetitive strain injury in secretaries: 340 secretaries, 65 with repetitive strain injury

8. Calculate the annual incidence of

 a. Work-related injuries in a car factory: 680 workers, four injuries per month
 b. Leukaemias in primary school children in a town near a nuclear energy plant, town population: 32 000; number of primary school children: 5800; number of leukaemia cases reported per year: 46

9. Calculate the age-specific mortality rate for the over-65-year age group in England: mid-year population for over 65 years is 9.2 million of which 30 914 died in one year

10. The prevalence of a disease

 a. Can only be calculated by a cohort study
 b. Is the number of new cases per unit time in a defined population
 c. Describes the balance between incidence, mortality and recovery
 d. Can be standardized for age and sex
 e. Can be used to compare the burden of a disease across different geographical areas

NHS, National Health Service; RSI, repetitive strain injury

EXPLANATION: MEASURING DISEASE

Disease occurrence can be measured in different ways and using different sources. One example is that of routinely collected data, i.e. data collected not for the specific purpose of conducting an epidemiological study, which can give estimates of the prevalence and incidence of a disease in a population.

1. **Denominator data (defining 'at risk' populations):** census

2. **Numerator data (defining cases)** – falls into several categories:
- **Mortality:** e.g. death registers and certificates
- **Morbidity:** e.g. NHS contact or disease registers
- **Wider impact:** e.g. cost to the NHS or days missed from work for health reasons.

3. **Prevalence** is the number of cases in a population at a single point in time divided by the total number of individuals in that population at the same point in time **(6)**. Prevalence is often expressed as a percentage (%) but for rarer diseases it can be expressed in larger population units such as per 1000 population or per 10 000 population.

The prevalence of disease at any time is determined by the incidence of new disease, the duration of the disease and changes in the population at risk, e.g. births and deaths. Prevalence measures the overall disease burden in a population at a particular point in time.

4. **Incidence** measures the number of **new** cases occurring in a defined time period divided by the number in the population at risk of becoming a case **(6)**. To estimate incidence, one needs:
- A defined population at risk of an event
- A defined time period
- The number of events occurring in that period.

Incidence is often considered by epidemiologists to be the most informative measure of disease occurence. It is expressed as the number of events per 1000 or per 100 000 population. For example, it is easier to think in terms of 12 deaths per 1000 than 0.012 deaths per person. The denominator for incidence can be refined and measured using 'person-time', e.g. person-years at risk, and this measure is often called the '**incidence rate**'.

Answers

6. See explanation

7. a – 38/170; 22 per cent; 22 smokers per 100 students, b – 65/340; 19 per cent; 19 per 100 secretaries get RSI

8. a – Injuries per year = 4 × 12 = 48; 48/680 = 0.07; 7 injuries per 100 workers per year, b – 46 cases per year/5800 primary school children = 0.0079; 79 leukaemia cases per 10 000 primary school children per year

9. 30 914/9 200 000 = 0.0034; 34 deaths per 10 000 population per year in the over-65-year age group

10. F F T T T

11. Which of the study designs are being described in the examples?

Options

A. Cohort study   C. Case–control study   E. Randomized controlled trial
B. Meta-analysis   D. Ecological study   F. Cross-sectional study

1. A group of Gulf War veterans is followed over the course of 10 years to determine the association between the exposure to life-threatening experiences and the risk of psychiatric disturbance
2. The prevalence of HIV is compared in two African countries, one with a national 'safe-sex' education programme in place and the other with no such programme
3. A group of patients with liver disease is questioned on its daily consumption of alcohol over the past year. Consumption rates are compared to those of a group of patients in the same hospital but without liver disease
4. Thirty women with breast cancer are given a new drug treatment and 30 similar women are given an existing treatment. Neither the doctors involved in the care of the women nor the women themselves are aware of which treatment they are taking. The women are followed over a period of five years and at the end the five-year survival rates for the two groups of women are calculated and compared
5. The prevalence of leukaemia in children living near power lines is compared with the prevalence in children living far away from power lines
6. All the existing evidence for the effectiveness of a new laparoscopic technique for resection of large bowel tumours from multiple different studies is collected together

12. Match the study designs below to the following scenarios (each option can be used once, more than once or not at all)

Options

A. Cohort study   C. Case–control study   E. Randomized controlled trial
B. Meta-analysis   D. Ecological study   F. Cross-sectional study

1. A rare disease
2. A rare risk factor
3. More than one outcome
4. Multiple risk factors
5. The temporal relationship between a risk factor and a disease
6. To prove the effect of a new drug for asthma
7. To test the hypothesis that hypertension is a risk factor for cardiovascular disease
8. When time and money are limited

HIV, human immunodeficiency virus

EXPLANATION: MEASURING ASSOCIATIONS

Special studies are used to assess the effects of exposure to particular risk or protective factors on a particular health outcome, such as a disease of interest.

The choice of a particular study design may depend upon a number of factors such as the prevalence of the condition of interest, the frequency of the exposure of interest or the amount of time and money available.

The table below summarizes the key characteristics, uses and disadvantages of the main types of epidemiological study.

Approach	Category	Type	Timing	Uses	Problems
Observational	Ecological study	Study of groups or populations using routinely collected data	Usually retrospective	Data on distribution of disease across population groups	No data about individuals
Observational	Cross-sectional study	Special health survey of individuals	One point in time	To measure prevalence	No incidence
Observational	Case–control study	Longitudinal study of individuals	Retrospective	For common exposure and rare outcome. Quick and cheap	Recall and selection bias. No proof of temporal relationship
Observational	Cohort study	Longitudinal study of individuals	Prospective or retrospective (historical data)	For rare exposures. Demonstrates a temporal relationship. Can measure incidence	Large sample sizes needed. Time consuming
Intervention	Randomized controlled trial	Clinical trial	Prospective	Gold standard for proving effect of an intervention	Expensive. Time consuming
Overview	Meta-analysis	Statistical review of numerical results of other studies	Retrospective	Summarizes all relevant research	Hard to include all published and unpublished data

Answers

11. 1 – A, 2 – D, 3 – C, 4 – E, 5 – F, 6 – B
12. 1 – C, 2 – A, 3 – A, 4 – C, 5 – AE, 6 – BE, 7 – A, 8 – BDF

SECTION 2

OBSERVATIONAL STUDIES: ECOLOGICAL STUDIES

OBSERVATIONAL STUDIES: ECOLOGICAL STUDIES

Seagroatt V. MMR vaccine and Crohn's disease: ecological study of hospital admissions in England, 1991 to 2002. *BMJ* 2005;330:1120–1121 (extracts and figures reproduced with permission from BMJ Publishing Group).

INTRODUCTION

'It has been hypothesised that the measles, mumps, and rubella vaccine (MMR vaccine) increases the risk of autism and Crohn's disease. Although a possible link with autism has been extensively studied and refuted, a link with Crohn's disease has not. I tested this hypothesis by analysing trends in age specific admission rates for Crohn's disease in children and adolescents to determine if the introduction of MMR vaccine in 1988 increased rates in those populations that were offered the vaccine as infants.'

1. What is the question being investigated by this study?

2. What type of comparison is being performed?

3. What types of data are being used to answer the question?

RESULTS

'Age specific rates per 10 000 population per year for emergency hospital admissions for Crohn's disease in England, 1991 to 2002. Rates in children aged < 4 years were relatively low and so were excluded from the figure. Three-year groups, rather than the more conventional five-year groups, were used in order to discriminate between rates in children born before and after the introduction of MMR.'

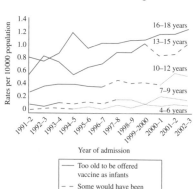

Year of admission

—— Too old to be offered vaccine as infants

– – Some would have been offered vaccine as infants

······ All would have been offered vaccine as infants

'There were 4463 admissions for Crohn's disease, 923 of which occurred in populations with a vaccination rate of ≥ 84 per cent (those born in 1988–89 or later). Although the age specific rates increased over the study period, no obvious changes occurred that coincided with the introduction of MMR vaccine. The estimated rate ratio for the MMR vaccination programme (rates in populations with a vaccination rate of ≥ 84 per cent compared with those with a rate of ≤ 7 per cent) was 0.95 (95 per cent confidence interval 0.84 to 1.08).'

4. What can we infer from the rate ratio and the confidence interval?

5. What potential confounding factors may influence the results?

MMR, measles, mumps and rubella

EXPLANATION: ECOLOGICAL STUDIES

In an **ecological study** the units of observation are populations or groups of people, rather than individuals. For example, an individual does not have a life expectancy or an income distribution, but a population of a city, state or country does. Ecological studies allow statements to be made about the populations being compared. While they may suggest associations between a disease and exposure, these usually require confirmation from studies involving individuals.

For **data collection**, disease rates and exposure are measured in each of a series of populations and their relationship is analysed. Ecological studies often use routinely collected aggregate statistics, usually published for other purposes, such as mortality rates or hospital admissions rates.

Populations can be compared in a variety of different ways:
- **Geographical comparison:** comparison of disease rates and prevalence of risk factors in different geographical areas
- **Temporal comparison:** ecological studies can be used to analyse trends in disease patterns over time by taking routinely collected statistics from the same population group over successive time intervals
- **Migrant studies:** the study of migrant populations helps to disentangle the influence of genetics and environmental exposures in determining disease processes. It can also help to establish the age at which environmental influences exert their effect. For example, studies looking at multiple sclerosis prevalence in migrant populations have shown that populations from places close to the equator maintain their low prevalence rates when they migrate to higher latitudes. However the offspring of the migrants adopt the high prevalence rates associated with the higher latitude location
- **Occupation and socio-economic group:** statistics on exposure and disease are widely available for specific groups in society. For example, occupational risk factors, such as the stress associated with working in the medical profession can be correlated with morbidity statistics such as rates of alcoholism in doctors.

The question being asked in the example study (page 12) is: 'Is there an association between the rate of Crohn's disease in children and the introduction of the MMR vaccine in 1988?' The study is a temporal comparison (1,2). The data used in the study come from two sources of **population-level data (3)**:

1. Routinely collected statistics for the age-specific rates of emergency hospital admissions for Crohn's disease for children under the age of 18 years from April 1991 to March 2003

2. Percentages of children completing a **primary course of MMR vaccine** in their second year of life (in the first two years of the MMR vaccination programme, these were 7 per cent and 68 per cent; thereafter they were at least 84 per cent).

Continued on page 16

Answers

1. See explanation
2. See explanation
3. See explanation
4. See explanation (page 16)
5. See explanation (page 16)

6. **Which one of the following definitions best describes the 'ecological fallacy'?**

   a. The weakness of ecological studies compared to case–control or cohort studies
   b. The mistaken interpretation of a study as ecological when really it is a cross-sectional study
   c. An association found in an ecological study does not exist at the individual level

7. **What are the advantages of an ecological study?**

   a. It can be used to study associations at the individual level
   b. It can study large and very different population groups
   c. It does not rely on existing published statistics which may contain errors
   d. It uses aggregate data on exposure and disease in population groups, increasing the power of the study
   e. It helps to formulate hypotheses on aetiological factors in disease
   f. It is easy to minimize confounding factors

8. **What are the disadvantages of an ecological study?**

   a. It cannot make inferences about individuals
   b. There is a risk of the ecological fallacy
   c. It is costly and time consuming to conduct
   d. It is less reliable than a case–control study that lacks within-population exposure variability
   e. It cannot compare populations that have very different characteristics

EXPLANATION: ADVANTAGES AND DISADVANTAGES OF ECOLOGICAL STUDIES

Advantages of an ecological study are:
- It is **quick, simple and cheap to conduct** due to the availability of routinely collected data that have already been published
- It has **more power than individual-level studies,** such as case–control and cohort studies where there is less exposure variability
- **Data can be used to compare populations with widely differing characteristics,** for example the Chinese and the Americans
- It **provides a useful starting point for more detailed epidemiological work** by helping to formulate hypotheses about the aetiology of disease.

Disadvantages are:
- The **risk of the 'ecological fallacy'**. This is when inappropriate conclusions are drawn on the basis of ecological data. An association seen at the group level does not necessarily represent an association at the individual level, therefore an ecological study cannot make inferences about individual level associations
- **Inability to control potential confounding factors other than age and sex.** For example, in geographical comparisons, although it may be possible to adjust for age and sex, data for other potential confounders, such as dietary or cultural habits, may not be available. In temporal studies, changes in diagnostic or treatment techniques may influence disease statistics over time. In migration studies, factors associated with the act of migration itself, such as psychological stress, may influence disease processes, confounding the influence of new environmental risk factors. In occupational studies, socio-economic factors may confound the results and vice versa
- **Reliance upon existing published statistics** may limit the breadth and type of studies conducted.

EXPLANATION: ECOLOGICAL STUDIES Cont'd from page 13

The **analysis** of data from ecological studies depends upon the mode of comparison being used, for example in geographical studies, associations between disease occurrence and exposure are often presented graphically in the form of scatter plots (see page 75). For temporal comparisons, **trends** may also be displayed graphically, and **correlation coefficients** (see page 107) or **rate ratios with confidence intervals** (as in the example study on page 12 and also see page 89) may be calculated.

A rate ratio of 0.95 suggests that the rate of emergency Crohn's admissions in children born after the introduction of the MMR vaccine (population group with $\geq$ 84 per cent vaccinated) is almost the same as the rate in the group born before the vaccine was introduced ($\leq$ 7 per cent vaccinated). The narrow confidence interval (which includes the value of 1) indicates that the rate ratio estimate is precise: we can be 95 per cent certain that the true rate ratio being estimated lies in the range 0.84 to 1.08 **(4)**.

Potential **confounders** (see page 117) could include **changes in dietary habit**, **new medical treatments** or another **immunological-type** factor with a protective effect against Crohn's disease in order to counteract an added risk from the MMR **(5)**. However, quoting from the example study: '. . . some factor(s) would have to be negatively associated with Crohn's disease, be introduced over the same three-year period, and be targeted at the same population of infants as MMR vaccine to mask a true association. This seems highly unlikely.'

MMR, measles, mumps and rubella.

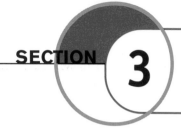

OBSERVATIONAL STUDIES: CROSS-SECTIONAL STUDIES

Chinn S and Rona RJ. Prevalence and trends in overweight and obesity in three cross sectional studies of British children, 1974–94. *BMJ* 2001;322:24–26 (summary of study reproduced with permission from the BMJ Publishing Group).

Study participants were primary school children, 10 414 boys and 9737 girls in England and 5385 boys and 5219 girls in Scotland aged 4 to 11 years. The height and body mass of all the children were measured and body mass index (BMI) calculated as weight/height^2, where weight was measured in kg and height in m.

Using linear interpolation between cut-off points for each six months of age, the percentages of children who were overweight or obese, as defined by the International Obesity Task Force (internationally agreed cut-off points equivalent to BMIs of 25 and 30 respectively at age 18 years) were calculated.

1. **Answer the following questions with reference to the above study:**

   a. What are the research questions being asked in this cross-sectional study?
   b. What features of the study design characterize it as cross-sectional?
   c. What type of data does it generate?
   d. What are the advantages and disadvantages of conducting the study in England and Scotland?

2. **From data in the table below, which shows a summary of results for 1974, what statements are correct regarding overweight and obesity in the UK?**

	Percentage prevalence of overweight children in 1974	Percentage prevalence of obese children in 1974
English boys	6.4	1.4
English girls	9.1	1.5
Scottish boys	5.4	1.7
Scottish girls	8.8	1.9

   a. The incidence of obesity is higher than the incidence of being overweight
   b. Girls and boys have a similar risk of being overweight
   c. The dietary habits of the Scots explain the higher rates of obesity in Scotland
   d. Nearly one in ten primary school-aged girls in England are considered overweight as defined by the International Obesity Task Force

---

BMI, body mass index

EXPLANATION: CROSS-SECTIONAL STUDIES (i)

A **cross-sectional study** usually involves a health survey of a group of **individuals** in a specified population **(1b)**. This is in contrast to an ecological study which uses routinely collected data about **groups**. Cross-sectional studies are particularly useful for estimating the prevalence of a condition or characteristic in a population, where the condition is a disease status defined in a standard way. These studies are conducted at a **single point in time** or over a **very short time period (1b)**, and are therefore unable to measure disease incidence. **Prevalence data rely upon strict definitions.** The definition of a disease state will influence prevalence data collected in a cross-sectional study. Taking the example opposite, different cut-off values of BMI would produce different prevalence estimates for obesity.

The validity of the prevalence data obtained from cross-sectional studies depends on **study participants** providing a **representative sample** of the relevant population. When the aim is to measure disease prevalence according to presence or absence of an exposure, they are not picked according to whether they have a disease or condition, or according to their exposure to any postulated factor **(1c)**. The number of 'cases' studied is therefore not specified in advance but is simply the number present in the sample. The best studies are those in which the participants are selected by a random method, for example from the electoral roll, school registers or general practitioners' lists, rather than by using volunteers **(1c)**. Non-random methods of recruiting participants, such as requesting volunteers or reliance on responses to postal questionnaires where the response rate is poor, may introduce bias into the sample population.

Cross-sectional studies can also be conducted simultaneously in different geographical places, so that prevalence can be compared in different areas. They may also compare different population groups, such as males versus females, different age groups, different socio-economic or ethnic groups. The questions asked in the example study are: 'What are the rates of obesity and overweight in the UK?' and 'Are there differences in prevalence between girls and boys/between England and Scotland/between age subgroups? **(1a)**'.

Advantages of conducting such a study in England and Scotland are that it is possible to obtain representative data for the whole of the UK and one can compare rates in different geographical areas to formulate hypotheses about causative environmental factors **(1d)**.

Disadvantages are that extra expense and co-ordination are needed to conduct more than one study simultaneously and there may be differences in methods of conducting the study in different geographical areas, leading to confounding factors **(1d)**.

This study is an example of a **descriptive** cross-sectional study. An **analytical** cross-sectional study collects data on both disease and exposure. Examples of analytical studies are:
• BRCA1 gene and diagnosis of breast cancer in women attending breast cancer screening clinics
• Prevalence of cancer in a representative sample of individuals in Chernobyl before and after the Chernobyl nuclear reactor disaster.

Answers

1. a – See explanation, b – See explanation, c – Prevalence data, d – See explanation
2. F F F T

Chinn S and Rona RJ. Prevalence and trends in overweight and obesity in three cross sectional studies of British children, 1974–94. *BMJ* 2001;322:24–26 (tables adapted with permission from the BMJ Publishing Group).

The example study described on page 18 was actually repeated at three sequential points in time, 1974, 1984 and 1994. Results are shown in the table below.

| | Change in prevalence of overweight (95 per cent CI) | |
	1974–84	1984–94
English boys	−1.0 (−2.1 to 0.1)	3.6 (2.3 to 5.0)
English girls	0.3 (−1.2 to 1.7)	4.1 (2.4 to 5.9)
Scottish boys	1.0 (−0.1 to 2.7)	3.6 (1.9 to 5.4)
Scottish girls	1.6 (−0.7 to 3.8)	5.4 (3.2 to 7.6)
	Change in prevalence of obesity (95 per cent CI)	
	1974–84	1984–94
English boys	−0.8 (−1.2 to −0.4)	1.2 (0.6 to 1.7)
English girls	−0.3 (−0.8 to 0.3)	1.4 (0.6 to 2.1)
Scottish boys	−0.8 (−1.7 to 0.0)	1.2 (0.5 to 2.0)
Scottish girls	−0.1 (−1.0 to 0.9)	1.4 (0.5 to 2.4)

3. **What do the results tell us about changes in prevalence of overweight children between 1974 and 1984, and 1984 and 1994?**

4. **How confident can we be in these results?**

5. **What conclusions can be drawn from the obesity data?**

6. **How could one improve the study, particularly regarding the obesity data?**

7. **What, if any, action would these results prompt you to take?**

CI, confidence interval

EXPLANATION: CROSS-SECTIONAL STUDIES (ii)

Cross-sectional studies are used to calculate the **prevalence** of a disease or condition at one particular point in time.

$$\text{Prevalence} = \frac{\text{Number of people with disease at a single point in time}}{\text{Total number studied at the same time point}}$$

However, cross-sectional studies can be repeated at different points in time to obtain sequential prevalence estimates and thus comment on trends in the population.

The example study tells us:

- **Overweight 1974 to 1984**: prevalence decreased in one group (English boys) but increased in others. In all groups the confidence interval includes 0, which means that one cannot exclude the possibility that there is no change in prevalence of overweight
- **Overweight 1984 to 1994**: prevalence in all groups has increased. This change is greatest in Scottish girls and the 95 per cent confidence intervals do not include 0 suggesting real increases
- **Obesity 1974 to 1984**: prevalence decreased in all groups. For English boys the estimated change in prevalence is –0.8 and the confidence interval does not include zero and suggests this is a real reduction
- **Obesity 1984 to 1994**: for all groups, the difference in prevalence shows an increase and the confidence intervals all exclude 0 suggesting this is a real increase **(3)**.

Confidence intervals (e.g. 95 per cent) can be calculated for changes in prevalence over time, providing a value for the statistical uncertainty associated with the estimated change in prevalence (see page 89). From the example given, the prevalence of overweight in English boys increased by 3.6 between 1984 and 1994 with a 95 per cent confidence interval of 2.3 to 5.0. This means that the true value of the increase in prevalence has a 95 per cent probability of being between 2.3 and 5.0 **(4)**. The prevalence changes for obesity are smaller. The estimated increase in prevalence in English boys between 1984 and 1994 was 1.2 with a 95 per cent confidence interval of 0.6 to 1.7. As this interval excludes zero we can conclude from these findings that there has been a real increase in obesity over the time frame investigated **(5)**.

The prevalence of obesity is much lower than that of overweight. The smaller number of cases reduces the statistical **precision of the study** for obesity. To increase the precision of obesity results, **the size of the study would need to be increased** (see pages 85 and 87) **(6)**.

The study has highlighted that the **prevalence of overweight in children is increasing** and suggests that there is a **similar rising trend** in the prevalence of obesity. Public health initiatives could be implemented for the **primary prevention** of overweight and for helping overweight children to maintain their weight, in order to prevent any further increases in the prevalence of obesity **(7)**.

Answers

3. See explanation
4. See explanation
5. See explanation
6. Increase sample size
7. See explanation

8. What are the advantages of a cross-sectional study?

    a. It is quick and inexpensive
    b. It can be used to calculate incidence
    c. It is good for studying common conditions
    d. It is good for looking at rare diseases
    e. It can be used to test a hypothesis
    f. It can be used to compare the prevalence data in different subsets of a population
    g. It can compare prevalence in populations in different geographical regions

9. Which of the following questions would be best investigated by using a cross-sectional study?

    a. Whether a new drug for hyperlipidaemia is effective at reducing serum triglyceride level
    b. Whether there is an association between obesity and childhood asthma
    c. Whether there has been a change in the incidence of heart disease in the under-40-year age group over the last 20 years
    d. Whether hay fever is more common in cities than rural areas
    e. Whether alcohol-related accidents are more common in France than in Britain

10. What are the disadvantages of a cross-sectional study?

    a. It cannot be used to estimate incidence
    b. There is a potential for recall bias
    c. Definitions of disease may influence prevalence estimates
    d. It can always demonstrate true trends in disease

11. In which of the following situations would a cross-sectional study be inappropriate?

    a. To test the hypothesis that obesity leads to an increased risk of asthma
    b. To calculate the number of new cases of obesity per year in the UK
    c. To study the prevalence of obesity in different countries of Europe
    d. To study whether the incidence of allergies changes with season
    e. To study whether exposure to mobile phone signals precedes development of brain tumours

BMI, body mass index

EXPLANATION: ADVANTAGES AND DISADVANTAGES OF CROSS-SECTIONAL STUDIES

Advantages of cross-sectional studies are:
- They are **relatively quick**: they are only conducted at a single point in time (unless a series of repeated studies is done) and therefore can be **relatively inexpensive**
- They can **give estimates of prevalence**
- They are **flexible**: they can be used for studying both rare and common conditions or diseases, depending on the sample size recruited
- They **can be used to compare prevalence in different populations and thus used to formulate hypotheses** about disease, based on characteristics such as sex, age or geographical location of a population
- **Sequentially repeated cross-sectional studies can be used to estimate changes in prevalence over time** and thus are used to demonstrate trends in health and disease.

Disadvantages of cross-sectional studies are:
- They **cannot measure incidence**: cross-sectional studies usually collect data only from a single point in time; including both new cases and those diagnosed in the past
- They **can be used to formulate but not formally test hypotheses regarding associations between subsequent disease following previous exposure**: the subjects are not chosen according to their exposure to a factor of interest or their disease status. It is only possible to use cross-sectional studies to study whether exposure and outcome may be associated. The results obtained may be interpreted in a number of different ways, giving rise to alternative explanations for the associations observed
- **Long-term outcomes**: cross-sectional studies do not provide information about the long-term outcomes of particular trends in health and disease status. Study participants are not followed up to a defined end-point and the consequences are not recorded, only the characteristic(s) of interest at the time of the survey. For example, the overweight and obesity study can only speculate on the future consequences of a trend of increasing BMI in children. It cannot provide hard proof as to the long-term medical complications of such a trend, as demonstrated by the following quote from the paper detailed on pages 18 and 20: 'Rising trends are *likely to be* reflected in increases in adult obesity and associated mortality'.

Answers
8. T F T F T T T
9. F T F T T
10. T F T F
11. T T F T T

OBSERVATIONAL STUDIES: CASE–CONTROL STUDIES

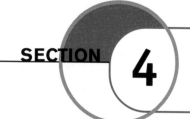

OBSERVATIONAL STUDIES: CASE–CONTROL STUDIES

Doll R and Hill AB. Smoking and carcinoma of the lung. Preliminary report. *BMJ* 1950;2:739–748 (extracts reproduced with permission from the BMJ Publishing Group).

'The great increase in the number of deaths attributed to cancer of the lung in the last 25 years justifies the search for a cause in the environment. An investigation was therefore carried out into the possible association of carcinoma of the lung with smoking, exposure to car and fuel fumes, occupation, etc. The preliminary findings with regard to smoking are reported.

'The material for the investigation was obtained from twenty hospitals in the London region which notified patients with cancer of the lung, stomach and large bowel. Almoners then visited and interviewed each patient. The patients with carcinoma of the stomach and large bowel served for comparison and, in addition, the almoners interviewed a non-cancer control group of general hospital patients, chosen so as to be of the same sex and age as the lung-carcinoma patients.'

---

1. Answer the following with reference to the above study:

    a. What question was this study designed to answer?
    b. What features of the study characterize it as a case–control study?
    c. What is the definition of a case in this study?
    d. Who are the controls?
    e. On what basis are cases and controls compared?
    f. What is the source population for the cases and controls?
    g. Can you think of any disadvantages of using this population as a source?
    h. How was information collected in this study?
    i. What are the disadvantages of using this method of data collection?

EXPLANATION: CASE–CONTROL STUDIES (i)

A **case–control study** is an observational epidemiological study where subjects are selected on the basis of whether they **have** (cases) or **do not have** (controls) a particular disease. A comparison is made between the proportion of subjects in the case and control groups who have been exposed to the aetiological factor under study. Case–control studies are always **retrospective**, i.e. they look back in time to determine past exposure in cases and controls **(1b)**.

The example study set out to answer the following question:
   'Is there an association between smoking and lung cancer?'; more precisely: 'Is it more likely that you were a smoker in the past if you have lung cancer now than if you don't have lung cancer now?'. In this study a 'case' is a person diagnosed with the disease of interest, i.e. a patient with lung cancer **(1a,1c)**.

'Controls' do not have lung cancer. They are not necessarily healthy – in this study, the controls had diseases such as cancer of the oesophagus or stomach, or non-cancer diseases not then thought to be associated with smoking **(1d)**. Cases and controls were compared with regard to their past smoking habits **(1e)**. The data were collected from patients from 20 London hospitals by personal interviews **(1f,1h)**. There are disadvantages of using patients only from London hospitals, as this may overlook other possible aetiological factors for lung cancer, such as pollution or overcrowding **(1g)**. Interviewers may consciously or subconsciously encourage particular answers or responders may not give accurate responses when asked questions face to face, introducing observer or responder bias, respectively **(1i)**.

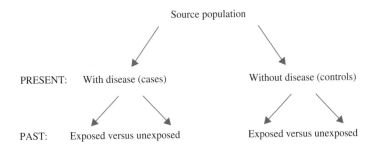

In a **matched study**, each case has one or more controls to which it is matched on an individual basis. Typical matching factors may include gender, age, occupation, region of residence, etc. The object of matching is to obtain a more accurate estimate of differences by 'removing' the possible influences of variables other than the exposure under investigation. The matching is done on confounding factors that are already established risk or protective factors, but are not under investigation themselves. There is a danger of over-matching, where cases and controls are matched on so many different confounding variables that it makes them over-similar with respect to potential aetiological factors of interest.

Answers
1. See explanation

Doll R and Hill AB. Smoking and carcinoma of the lung. Preliminary report. *BMJ* 1950;2:739–748 (table adapted with permission from the BMJ Publishing Group).

The table below shows results obtained from this study.

Patients	Total number of patients	Number who are smokers
Males		
Lung cancer	649	647
No lung cancer	649	622
Females		
Lung cancer	60	41
No lung cancer	60	28

2. Which method is commonly used to present the results of a case–control study?

3. Use this method for the above data on males and females

4. What measure of association is used to summarize the results of a case–control study?

5. Calculate the value of this measure of association for the above data

6. Comment on the meaning of these calculated values

7. State the null hypothesis for a case–control study

8. What simple hypothesis test can be applied to the results of a case–control study?

9. Apply this test to the above data

10. What value is calculated to determine the statistical significance of the test statistic?

11. Why does this value differ for men and women?

CI, confidence interval; OR, odds ratio

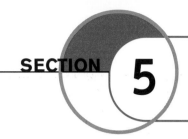

OBSERVATIONAL STUDIES: COHORT STUDIES

Song Y-M, Sung J, Lawlor DA *et al*. Blood pressure, haemorrhagic stroke, and ischaemic stroke: the Korean national prospective occupational cohort study. *BMJ* 2004;328:324–325 (extracts reproduced with permission from BMJ Publishing Group).

'We examined the association of blood pressure with subtype of stroke in a large cohort of Korean civil servants. Blood pressure was measured for individuals between 1986 and 1996 during their biennial health examinations. We included deaths attributed to all strokes, haemorrhagic and ischaemic between 1991 and 2000 in these analyses. We categorized non-fatal strokes using data on the use of medical care, and found an accuracy of 83.4 per cent and 85.7 per cent for ischaemic stroke and haemorrhagic stroke.

'In 9.5 million person years of observation of 955 271 people; they had 14 057 strokes, giving crude and age standardized incidences of 1.48 and 2.24 for every 1000 person years. Of these, 10 716 (76 per cent) strokes had complete information on major exposure variables and we included these in our analyses; we classified 2695 strokes as haemorrhagic, 5326 as ischaemic, 1731 as undetermined, and 964 as subarachnoid haemorrhage.

'Multiple characteristics were measured as variables that are known or potential risk factors for ischaemic or haemorrhagic strokes. These included age, sex, body mass index (BMI), height, blood glucose, blood cholesterol, haemoglobin concentration, ethanol consumption, smoking, monthly pay level, and area of residency.

'We calculated fully adjusted relative risks and 95 per cent confidence intervals using logistic regression. . . . Both ischaemic stroke and haemorrhagic stroke had strong gradients with blood pressure, but these were much steeper for haemorrhagic stroke. . . . For each higher 20 mmHg of systolic blood pressure, the relative risk of ischaemic and haemorrhagic stroke increased by 2.23 (2.17 to 2.30) and 3.18 (3.06 to 3.30), z test for difference between odds ratios 11.40, $P < 0.00001$. . . . Our findings emphasize the importance of controlling blood pressure, particularly in countries with a high risk of haemorrhagic stroke.'

---

1. **Answer the following with reference to the study above**

   a. What question has this study been designed to answer?
   b. What features of this study suggest that it is a cohort study?
   c. Is this a prospective or retrospective cohort study?
   d. What are the likely sources of error in this study?

BMI, body mass index

EXPLANATION: COHORT STUDIES (i)

A cohort study is a type of **observational** epidemiological study.

A cohort study can be either **prospective** (current) or **retrospective** (historical). In a prospective study, the data on exposure are collected prior to the occurrence of disease and subjects are followed up over time to observe occurrence of the disease. In a retrospective study, past exposure data are assembled for a defined cohort using historical records. The disease outcome may or may not be known at this time; ideally it should be obtained independent from or subsequent to assembly of exposure data.

The figure below gives a diagrammatic representation of different cohort study designs.

The example given is a huge prospective cohort study **(1c)** designed to investigate if there is any association between blood pressure and subtype of stroke (haemorrhagic or ischaemic) **(1a)**. The factors that made this typical of a cohort study were that a large 'cohort' of study participants was defined according to participants' exposure (high blood pressure) rather than according to their disease status, and that participants were followed over time to determine subsequent stroke risk **(1b)**.

A major **limitation of cohort studies**, particularly those done over a long time period, is loss of subjects due to factors such as death or migration. In this example, complete information was only collected on 76 per cent of recorded strokes, therefore almost a quarter of outcomes have not been related to exposure; this could be a potentially huge source of error, especially if relative risks were smaller. Some of the tools available to reduce error due to loss of subjects when analysing the results of a cohort study are discussed on page 39.

Likely sources of **error** in the study in question include bias, confounding, human error in measuring the initial blood pressures and error due to incomplete information **(1d)**.

Answers

1. See explanation

2. Using the results table opposite, answer the following true or false

a. You are less likely to have a stroke if you have normal blood pressure
b. If you have very high blood pressure you are almost 20 times as likely to have a fatal stroke than if you have normal blood pressure
c. If you have a very high blood pressure you are almost 20 times as likely to have an ischaemic stroke than if you have normal blood pressure
d. The larger the number (of people having strokes) the smaller the range of the confidence intervals

3. Using the results table on page 37 answer the following as percentages

a. What is the probability that less than 16.41 times as many people with very high blood pressure as normal blood pressure have a fatal stroke?
b. What is the probability that between 24.89 and 33.40 times as many people with very high blood pressure as normal blood pressure have a haemorrhagic stroke?

4. Choose from the following options the most appropriate test for the situations given

Options

A. Chi-squared tests (see page 122)
B. z-test for numeric data (see page 95)
C. Cox proportional hazards (see page 39)
D. Hypothesis testing (see page 93)
E. Calculating confidence intervals (see page 89)

1. Determining if results are statistically significant
2. Estimating the size of the effect on the outcome of the exposure
3. Comparing the means of continuous variables (height, BMI, age, etc.) in two groups
4. Comparing the dichotomous variables (male/female, etc.) in the groups
5. To account for differences other than exposure (blood pressure) or risk of outcome (stroke)

BMI, body mass index

EXPLANATION: COHORT STUDIES (ii)

The risk estimates obtained from this cohort study have been presented as relative risk rather than absolute values. See page 105 on **relative risk** and **absolute risk**. This is sometimes a useful way of representing the information as it can be seen at a glance that, whatever subcategory of stroke is considered, a given individual is between 8 and 34 times as likely to have a stroke if their blood pressure is very high.

The disadvantage of representing the data as relative risk values is that the absolute risk of ischaemic and haemorrhagic stroke in each of the blood pressure groups cannot be compared directly. The increase in relative risk of haemorrhagic stroke is much greater than the increase in relative risk of ischaemic stroke with increased blood pressure; 28.83 times compared to 9.56 times normal values, respectively. The absolute risk of an ischaemic stroke if one has very high blood pressure might still be higher than haemorrhagic stroke. This depends on the magnitude of the risk of each condition for those with normal blood pressure.

The best cohort studies will identify **potential confounding variables** and consider whether they differ between the two groups. If there are statistically significant differences, e.g. higher cholesterol levels in the very high blood pressure group, these can be adjusted for in the data analyses. In the example study, the confounding variables adjusted for included age, gender, BMI, height, blood glucose, blood cholesterol, haemoglobin concentration, ethanol consumption, smoking, monthly pay level, and area of residency.

The table below shows relative risks (95 per cent confidence intervals) for mean blood pressure from the Korean National Health System Study, 1986–2000.

	All strokes fatal	Non-fatal	Stroke subtypes Ischaemic	Haemorrhagic
Number of strokes	2073	8643	5326	2695
Blood pressure (mmHg)				
< 140/< 90 Normal	1	1	1	1
≥ 180/≥ 110 Very high	19.39 (16.41 to 22.90)	11.21 (10.17 to 12.36)	9.56 (8.46 to 10.80)	28.83 (24.89 to 33.40)

Song Y-M, Sung J, Lawlor DA *et al*. Blood pressure, haemorrhagic stroke, and ischaemic stroke: the Korean national prospective occupational cohort study. *BMJ* 2004;328:324–325 (table adapted with permission from the BMJ Publishing Group).

Answers

2. T T F T
3. a – 2.5 per cent, b – 95 per cent (look at the confidence intervals)
4. 1 – D, 2 – E, 3 – B, 4 – A, 5 – C

A group of 20 young adults went on a 2-week-long skiing trip. On the first day one person broke a finger and another broke an arm. On the third day someone tore a ligament in their knee; two further injuries occurred in the first week, one on the fifth day and one on the sixth day. On the penultimate day of the holiday one of the members of the group broke their leg. Each of the members of the group who was injured stopped skiing from the time they were injured onwards.

5. What is the risk, per day, of a skier in the group of 20 having an injury?

    a. On the first day
    b. If the holiday were only 1 week long
    c. Over the 2 weeks

6. What was the average number of days that each member of the group spent skiing during the 2-week holiday?

7. Which of the following compares 'time to event' in two groups?

    a. Log rank
    b. Cox proportional hazards
    c. Odds ratio
    d. Kaplan–Meier survival curves

8. The curve below showing the probability of survival tells us:

    a. Less than 25 per cent survive 5 years
    b. 75 per cent survive 10 years
    c. 90 per cent survive 5 years
    d. More than 50 per cent survive 10 years

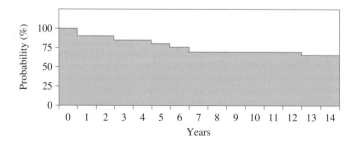

EXPLANATION: COHORT STUDIES (iii)

A **Kaplan–Meier survival curve** compares the prognosis of different conditions and different treatments used at different times, with different periods of follow-up. A survival curve allows us to estimate the cumulative probability of an event occurring, using data from the subjects who are still alive and available at the last follow-up. This allows us to calculate the expected time period for a particular event to occur. Although survival curves were originally used to assess mortality, they can be used to assess any outcome, for example, time for a fracture to heal, time to discontinuation of a psychiatric drug and many others.

An example survival curve for two childhood cancers is shown below.

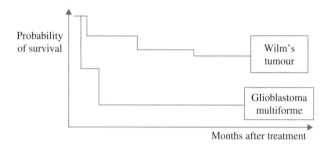

Each step on the curve represents the change in probability as individual events occur. For example, if two children out of 20 die between 2 and 6 weeks, the probability of survival will fall by 10 per cent over that 4-week interval. As the sample size increases, the steps will become smaller and closer together, smoothing out the curve.

The **Cox proportional hazard model** is a useful analytical tool in cohort studies as it helps reduce error due to loss to follow-up from deaths and dropout of subjects. Supposing that in the example study (page 34) all the people with very high blood pressure had their strokes in the first 2 years, while those with normal blood pressure had their strokes 7 or 8 years afterwards. The method used there (logistic regression) would not take this into account. It would then be more useful to compare the time between exposure (having high blood pressure) and the outcome (stroke).

The Cox proportional hazards model is the most widely used method of comparing 'time to event' in medical research. Other appropriate methods include **log rank** and the **Wilcoxon two-sample** tests **(7)**.

Answers

5. a – (2/20)/1= 10 per cent, b – (5/20)/7 = 3.6 per cent, c – (6/20)/14 = 2.1 per cent
6. Over the possible 280 days of skiing (20 × 14) only 225 were spent skiing. This is 11.25 days each
7. T T F T
8. F F F T

9. What are the advantages of a prospective cohort study?

    a. It is quick and inexpensive
    b. It can be used to determine the temporal relationship between risk factor and disease
    c. It is good for looking at rare diseases
    d. The outcome following rare exposures can be measured
    e. Information can be collected during the study and will not be biased by the outcome
    f. It can be used to calculate incidence

10. What are the disadvantages of a cohort study?

    a. Only one outcome can be measured
    b. The cohort may be a biased sample due to the health-related selection
    c. It is expensive and time consuming
    d. Only values for relative risk can be calculated

EXPLANATION: ADVANTAGES AND DISADVANTAGES OF COHORT STUDIES

Advantages of cohort studies are:
- They are longitudinal and, unless a retrospective study, exposure data can be collected from the start and throughout the course of the study. This permits the collection of complete, unbiased information about subjects' exposure before the outcome is known
- A more accurate conclusion of the **temporal relationship** between the exposure and the following incidence of disease can be drawn
- **Multiple outcomes** related to a specific or single exposure can be measured
- **Incidence rates** (absolute risk) can be calculated as well as relative risk
- They can be used to study the outcome of relatively **rare exposures**.

Disadvantages of cohort studies are:
- Difficulty with the method of selection. Often the way that people are enrolled in such studies is via advertising or choosing groups of people who present to healthcare services frequently. Some famous cohort studies have avoided this problem by recruiting all members of well-defined groups, such as physicians, civil servants or even medical students. There may, however, be problems in generalising the results obtained to the wider population. Initially participants are usually healthy, but over the course of a long study their health may deteriorate as part of a natural progression. This is sometimes referred to as health-related selection (see page 117 on bias)
- Cohort studies are not suitable for **rare disease** as a huge initial cohort would be needed. Large studies are **expensive** to carry out, follow-up appointments are **time consuming**, and a large team is usually involved in data collection
- **Loss to follow-up** such as migration or death is a huge disadvantage, and the longer the follow-up the greater the loss tends to be. If there is a high dropout rate (> 20 per cent), it becomes difficult to draw accurate conclusions
- Changes over time, such as advances in treatment, may vary exposure over the course of the study and make the results irrelevant
- Exposure may be linked to a **hidden confounder** that is not measured
- **Blinding is difficult** in cohort studies; if people know they have very high blood pressure this may have either a positive or negative effect on outcome. They may start to exercise, stop smoking or take medication, thus decreasing their risks, or conversely the added stress of knowing their risk is higher may become a confounding factor that increases their overall risk.

Specific advantages and **disadvantages** of **retrospective** cohort studies are:
- If the time taken from exposure to disease outcome is very long, a prospective cohort study may have a high dropout rate; an advantage of a retrospective cohort study is that it only includes subjects for whom complete data from exposure to outcome is available
- A disadvantage is there may be bias in measuring exposure when disease outcome is known.

Answers
9. F T F T T T
10. F T T F

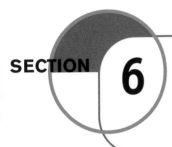

SECTION 6

INTERVENTION STUDIES: RANDOMIZED CONTROLLED TRIALS

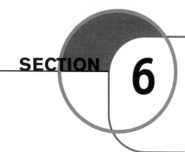

INTERVENTION STUDIES: RANDOMIZED CONTROLLED TRIALS

Ballard C, Margallo-Lana M, Juszczak E, *et al*. Quetiapine and rivastigmine and cognitive decline in Alzheimer's disease: randomised double blind placebo controlled trial. *BMJ* 2005; 330:874 (extracts reproduced with permission from the BMJ Publishing Group).

'Ninety-three patients with Alzheimer's disease, dementia, and clinically significant agitation were chosen from care facilities in the north east of England to determine the respective efficacy of quetiapine and rivastigmine for agitation in people with dementia in institutional care. The trial was also designed to evaluate these treatments with respect to change in cognitive performance.

'Patients were randomly sorted into three groups of equal numbers. Each group was assigned the atypical antipsychotic quetiapine plus a placebo, the cholinesterase inhibitor rivastigmine plus placebo, or placebo (double dummy) for 26 weeks. Agitation and cognition were measured at baseline and at six weeks and 26 weeks.

'Seventy-one (89 per cent) of the patients tolerated the maximum protocol dose (22 rivastigmine, 23 quetiapine, 26 placebo). Compared with placebo, neither group showed significant differences in improvement on the agitation inventory either at six weeks or 26 weeks. For quetiapine the change in cognitive score from baseline was estimated as an average of −14.6 points (95 per cent CI −25.3 to −4.0) lower than in the placebo group at six weeks ($P = 0.009$), and −15.4 points (−27.0 to −3.8) lower at 26 weeks ($P = 0.01$). The corresponding changes with rivastigmine were −3.5 points (−13.1 to 6.2) lower at six weeks ($P = 0.5$), and −7.5 points (−21.0 to 6.0) lower at 26 weeks ($P = 0.3$).

'Conclusion: Neither quetiapine nor rivastigmine are effective in the treatment of agitation in people with dementia in institutional care. Compared with placebo, quetiapine is associated with significantly greater cognitive decline.'

---

1. Answer the following with reference to the study above:

    a. What questions was this study designed to answer?
    b. What features of the design show it is a randomized controlled trial?
    c. Is it an observational or intervention study?
    d. What are the likely sources of error in this study?

---

2. The design features listed below reduce error in the study. True or False?

    a. Randomizing patients into treatment groups   **c.** Using placebo treatments
    b. The use of blinding   **d.** The use of double blinding

---

CI, confidence interval

EXPLANATION: RANDOMIZED CONTROLLED TRIALS (i)

Randomized controlled trials are considered the '**gold standard**' of clinical and epidemiological studies. They are **intervention** studies that choose a group of patients who are suitable for one or more types of drug or intervention (e.g. surgery). If one treatment is being tested then it can be compared with either placebo or the existing gold standard. Further comparisons may be made between treatments or population subtypes by addition of 'arms' to the trial. Additionally, more than one treatment or combinations of treatments could be compared directly to **placebo**. A conclusion drawn from a carefully conducted randomized controlled trial that is of adequate size and has used techniques such as **double blinding** or placebo treatments is considered the most reliable, sometimes referred to as 'top level' or 'level 1', evidence as to whether a treatment is effective or not.

The example on page 44 is an intervention study (**1c**) to compare quetiapine, rivastigmine and a placebo with respect to (a) levels of agitation, and (b) decline in cognition in patients with Alzheimer's disease, dementia and agitation (**1a**). Patients were assigned to one treatment group at random: quetiapine plus placebo, rivastigmine plus placebo or placebo only (**1b**). The likely sources of error in the study arise mainly from small treatment groups and that anxiety and cognition are inherently difficult to assess (**1d**).

In the best studies all patients are suitable for each of the options, and **randomization** is done using 'names out of a hat' or random number generation. Generally the aim is for there to be equal numbers in each group. With a large enough trial, random allocation should lead to a very similar distribution of characteristics in each group (mean age, male to female ratio, etc).

Blinding can be single, where either the patient or the doctor is unaware of which treatment has been given; or it can be double in which case neither the patient nor the doctor knows which treatment is being given. In the example given, double blinding was carried out: 'The randomizing clinician faxed a form to the statistician, who communicated allocation to the pharmacy, ensuring concealment.' The term 'double blinding' may be misleading, as often more than two people in the study are blinded, for example the statisticion performing the analysis may be blinded as well as the doctor and patient.

In **crossover** trials comparisons are not made between patients but within patients when, over a period of time, each patient receives more than one treatment. Each patient is randomly assigned to one treatment 'arm' involving a sequence of two or more interventions given consecutively. One example is that of an AB/BA study, where A and B may be types of drug or treatment, or one a treatment and the other a placebo. In the first round, half of the group is randomly assigned to A, while the other half is randomly assigned to B. After a 'dry out' period the two groups swap. This has the advantage of comparing each subject's response to both treatments and also reveals if the order of treatment has an effect.

Sometimes the effect measured when a patient thinks they are on treatment is significant, this is known as the **placebo effect**. If part of the group is randomized to 'no treatment', they will be given an identical looking placebo tablet and contact time with health professionals will be the same.

Answers
1. See explanation
2. T T T T

3. The following are advantages of having a large sample

a. More data for statistical comparison
b. It is cheap and easy to perform a trial on large numbers of people
c. A large initial sample allows for there to be enough data once non-compliance has been taken into account

4. What are the disadvantages of having a large sample?

a. It is easier to make type 1 and type 2 errors (see page 113)
b. It is ethically wrong to treat a lot of people with a substandard treatment that can be proved so by exposing far fewer people
c. Even though the conclusions are statistically significant they are weak

5. Using the compliance adjustment formula, adjust the calculated sample size per arm $(N) = 100$ for a trial that expects 80 per cent compliance ($c = 0.8$) in each group

Ballard C, Margallo-Lana M, Juszczak E, *et al.* Quetiapine and rivastigmine and cognitive decline in Alzheimer's disease: randomised double blind placebo controlled trial. *BMJ* 2005; 330:874 (extract reproduced with permission from the BMJ Publishing Group).

The following explains how the sample size was chosen:
'To detect an average difference of a 6-point (SD 6) change in agitation inventory score from baseline to six weeks between active treatment and placebo with a power of 90 per cent at the 5 per cent (two sided) level of significance, we needed a sample size of 23 in each group, assuming similar efficacy of active treatments. These parameters are based on the effect reported for carbamazepine in a similar study. With allowance for a drop out rate of 25 per cent, we therefore needed 31 patients per treatment group ($n = 93$).'

6. In the example above how does the non-compliance affect the sample size?

a. If the non-compliance was 20 per cent how many patients per group would have been needed?
b. If the non-compliance was 30 per cent how many patients per group would have been needed?
c. If the power was 95 per cent at the 2.5 per cent level of significance would this require a larger or smaller sample?

SD, standard deviation

EXPLANATION: RANDOMIZED CONTROLLED TRIALS (ii)

There are several important reasons to get the sample size right. Firstly the **numbers need to be big enough** so that if the treatment really does affect clinical outcome, the trial will be able to detect a statistically significant difference. However, the bigger the sample size, the **more time and money** the trial will cost. Randomized controlled trials may be designed as large-scale, multicentre trials if two very similar treatments are being compared and the difference between them cannot be determined by smaller studies. From an **ethical** perspective, the closer the two treatments are to each other, or indeed to the 'gold standard', the more reasonable it is to involve hundreds or thousands of people in the trial.

This is a checklist devised for working out how big the sample size should be:
- Estimate the event rate in the control group by extrapolating from a population similar to the population enrolled in the trial
- Determine the smallest difference that will be of clinical importance
- Determine the power (see page 115) for the particular trial
- Determine the significance level or probability of a type 1 error (see page 115) that is acceptable or reasonable (see page 97 on significance levels and *P*-values)
- Adjust the calculated sample size (*N*) for the expected dropout rate or level of non-compliance with treatment.

The level of **non-compliance** takes into account the proportion of patients allocated to treatment who fail to take it as well as those on placebo who do end up on treatment. A placebo-controlled study needing 100 patients per treatment arm, with 100 per cent compliance, would require over 278 patients per arm if compliance were only 80 per cent in each group. If compliance fell to 70 per cent in each group, the trial would require 625 patients.

The compliance adjustment formula is as follows: Adjusted n per arm $= \dfrac{N}{(c_1 + c_2 - 1)^2}$ where c_1 and c_2 are the average compliance or inverse dropout rates per arm.

The figure opposite depicts the exponential increase in numbers needed in the initial sample as the dropout rate or non-compliance increases. The three different lines represent compliance of 70 per cent, 80 per cent and 90 per cent respectively in the control group.

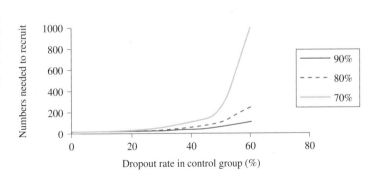

7. What are the advantages of randomized controlled trials?

    a. They can study an intervention for which there is no observational information
    b. Large trials are cheap and easy to organize
    c. They can be designed with features to eliminate bias

8. What are the disadvantages of randomized controlled trials?

    a. They are not considered very highly as a type of epidemiological study
    b. By randomizing the subjects the study is open to bias
    c. Blinding can cause ethical problems

9. How might study design take advantages and disadvantages into account?

10. Put the options in the order that would suggest 'goodness' of study design from the worst to the best, assuming each feature is both possible and appropriate

Options

    A. Non-randomized
    B. Randomized, placebo, crossover and double blinding
    C. Randomized, placebo, crossover and single blinding
    D. Randomized
    E. Randomized, placebo and crossover
    F. Randomized with placebo

EXPLANATION: META-ANALYSIS (ii)

To perform an effective meta-analysis:
- **Evaluate the results from individual studies.** Ideally look at the raw data but if this is not available for each study, results can be assessed using published results
- **Estimate the degree of variability in the results between studies.** This variability is known as the 'statistical heterogeneity'
- **Obtain a numerical estimate for the average effect by combining results from all the studies.** When comparing studies the 'size of the effect' should be comparable, and will often be expressed as an odds ratio, a relative risk or a standardized mean difference
- **Determine the strength and significance of the overall effect** by obtaining a 95 per cent or 99 per cent confidence interval and performing a hypothesis test
- **Present the findings.** This is commonly done using a graphical display known as a **forest plot**. This shows the estimated effect size, such as relative risk or risk ratio, obtained from each contributing study. Each relative risk estimate is plotted using a square shape, where the size of the square is proportional to the size of the study. In general, the larger the study, the larger the square used to represent the estimate from that study. Confidence intervals for each estimate are also plotted, as shown in the figure below. Forest plots also show the overall estimate obtained from analyses of results from all studies combined. This overall estimate is indicated by a diamond shape near the bottom of the graph. Here the length of the diamond indicates the width of the confidence interval for the overall estimate.

The forest plot allows readers to find quickly the answer to the following questions:
- Is the effect from each study on the same side of the vertical line?
- How precise are the results from each study, i.e. the width of each confidence interval?
- Are the results from the different studies compatible, i.e. do the confidence intervals overlap?
- Is the effect significant? Do confidence intervals cross the vertical line?

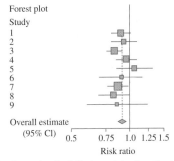

Forest plot

Graph reproduced wth kind permission from Everitt BS and Palmer CR (eds), *Encydopaedic Companion to Medical Statistics*, Great Britain: Hodder Education, 2005

Whether or not these results would lead to a change in a doctor's clinical practice is a subjective matter **(6)**. Quoting from the conclusion of the study (page 54):
> 'Increased risks of suicide and self harm caused by SSRIs cannot be ruled out, but larger trials with longer follow up are required to assess the balance of risks and benefits fully. Any such risks should be balanced against the effectiveness of SSRIs in treating depression.'

Since there is no definite evidence either way to say that SSRIs increase the risks of suicide, the study recommends:
> 'When prescribing SSRIs, clinicians should warn patients of the possible risk of suicidal behaviour and monitor patients closely in the early stages of treatment.' **(7)**.

Answers

5. a – No increased risk of suicide (OR = 0.85, CI includes the value of 1), b – A slight increase in the risk of self-harm (OR = 1.57, CI > 1), c – No increased risk of suicidal thoughts (OR = 0.77, CI includes the value of 1)

6. See explanation

7. See explanation

8. Which of the following are advantages of meta-analysis?

    a. Less power

    b. Smaller sample size needed

    c. Generation of new data

    d. More precise

9. Which of the following are possible disadvantages of meta-analysis?

    a. Dependence on publication

    b. Costly

    c. Loss to follow-up

    d. Risk of excluding unpublished data

    e. Incompatibility between component study designs

10. Match up the advantages to the study designs from the options given

Options

    A. Ecological study

    B. Cross-sectional study

    C. Case–control study

    D. Cohort study

    E. Randomized controlled trial

    F. Meta-analysis

    1. Can compare widely differing populations

    2. Can provide an estimate of relative risk

    3. Can summarize results of all the studies asking a similar question

    4. Can demonstrate a temporal relationship between exposure to a risk factor and development of disease

    5. Can directly measure the effects of an intervention

    6. Can estimate prevalence

11. Match up the following diasdvantages to the study designs from the options given

Options

    A. Ecological study

    B. Cross-sectional study

    C. Case–control study

    D. Cohort study

    E. Randomized controlled trial

    F. Meta-analysis

    1. Risk of loss to follow-up

    2. Cannot make inferences about individual-level risks

    3. Cannot estimate incidence

    4. Cannot prove the existence of a temporal relationship between risk factor and effect

    5. May mask heterogeneity between individual studies and thus produce an invalid conclusion

    6. Expensive and time consuming

EXPLANATION: ADVANTAGES AND DISADVANTAGES OF META-ANALYSIS

Advantages of meta-analysis are:
- **Condenses large amounts of information** into managable portions
- **Greater power and precision** to detect an effect than the individual component studies, due to its larger sample size
- **Faster and cheaper** than performing a whole new study
- **Avoids unnecessary repetition** of previous studies
- **Can be used to generalize results** to a wider population
- Can be **used to assess consistency** between studies
- **Permits assessment of the quality of existing evidence** and identifies outstanding research questions to be addressed
- **May help to resolve conflicts or uncertainties** in original trials
- **May be the study of choice** if it is not practical or ethical to conduct a definitive trial.

Disadvantages of meta-analysis are:
- **Publication bias**: some data may not have been published if the results were insignificant. A full meta-analysis should identify unpublished as well as published studies to provide a non-biased review
- **Inconsistency between studies** in characteristics such as patient population, methodology, outcome measures and follow-up procedure may mean that the results of the different studies cannot be compared directly
- **Studies may differ in the quality of their design**. Although this should be accounted for by weighting, the weighting value may be subjective and arbitrary
- **Dependence**: the results of one study may be published more than once, and therefore the data from different studies in the meta-analysis may not be entirely independent
- **Important qualitative information may be obscured** by 'averaging' simple numerical representations across studies. This is especially the case if there are two outcomes or a bimodal population.

Answers

8. F F F T
9. T F F T T
10. 1 – A, 2 – C, 3 – F, 4 – D, 5 – E, 6 – B
11. 1 – D, 2 – A, 3 – B, 4 – C, 5 – F, 6 – E

Gunnell D, Saperia J and Ashby D. Selective serotonin reuptake inhibitors (SSRIs) and suicide in adults: meta-analysis of drug company data from placebo controlled, randomised controlled trials submitted to the MHRA's safety review. *BMJ* 2005;330:385 (graphs reproduced with permission from the BMJ Publishing Group).

Forest plots of suicide, non-fatal self-harm and suicidal thoughts in placebo controlled trials of SSRIs.

(a) Meta-analysis of suicide data[1]

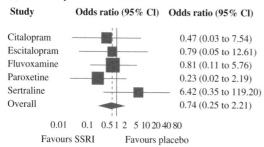

Study		Odds ratio (95% CI)
Citalopram		0.47 (0.03 to 7.54)
Escitalopram		0.79 (0.05 to 12.61)
Fluvoxamine		0.81 (0.11 to 5.76)
Paroxetine		0.23 (0.02 to 2.19)
Sertraline		6.42 (0.35 to 119.20)
Overall		0.74 (0.25 to 2.21)

(b) Meta-analysis of non-fatal self-harm data (excluding and including paroxetine)

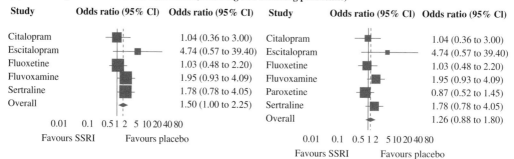

Excluding paroxetine:
Study	Odds ratio (95% CI)
Citalopram	1.04 (0.36 to 3.00)
Escitalopram	4.74 (0.57 to 39.40)
Fluoxetine	1.03 (0.48 to 2.20)
Fluvoxamine	1.95 (0.93 to 4.09)
Sertraline	1.78 (0.78 to 4.05)
Overall	1.50 (1.00 to 2.25)

Including paroxetine:
Study	Odds ratio (95% CI)
Citalopram	1.04 (0.36 to 3.00)
Escitalopram	4.74 (0.57 to 39.40)
Fluoxetine	1.03 (0.48 to 2.20)
Fluvoxamine	1.95 (0.93 to 4.09)
Paroxetine	0.87 (0.52 to 1.45)
Sertraline	1.78 (0.78 to 4.05)
Overall	1.26 (0.88 to 1.80)

(c) Meta-analysis of suicidal thoughts data (excluding and including paroxetine)

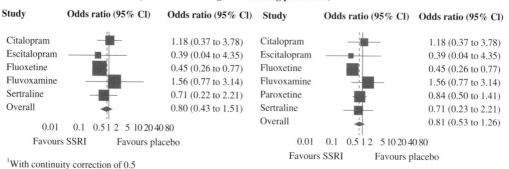

Excluding paroxetine:
Study	Odds ratio (95% CI)
Citalopram	1.18 (0.37 to 3.78)
Escitalopram	0.39 (0.04 to 4.35)
Fluoxetine	0.45 (0.26 to 0.77)
Fluvoxamine	1.56 (0.77 to 3.14)
Sertraline	0.71 (0.22 to 2.21)
Overall	0.80 (0.43 to 1.51)

Including paroxetine:
Study	Odds ratio (95% CI)
Citalopram	1.18 (0.37 to 3.78)
Escitalopram	0.39 (0.04 to 4.35)
Fluoxetine	0.45 (0.26 to 0.77)
Fluvoxamine	1.56 (0.77 to 3.14)
Paroxetine	0.84 (0.50 to 1.41)
Sertraline	0.71 (0.23 to 2.21)
Overall	0.81 (0.53 to 1.26)

[1]With continuity correction of 0.5

SSRI, selective serotonin reuptake inhibitor
In contrast with page 54, these plots show odds ratios with 95% confidence intervals (95% CI) calculated using a classical approach

DESCRIBING DATA

1. How would you display the following sets of data, choose from the options given

Options

A. Scatter plot   **B.** Pie chart   **C.** Histogram

1. The relationship between proximity to site of explosion and levels of contaminant in urine
2. The distribution of mean red blood cell volume
3. Causes of the wrong blood being transfused in patients in a UK hospital
4. The relationship between blood creatinine and urea levels in a series of patients
5. Causes of stroke by subtype
6. The distribution of weights of all the staff in a GP practice

2. Match the following distributions of data to how they should be represented graphically

Options

A. J-shaped   **B.** Skewed to right (positive)   **C.** Skewed to left (negative)   **D.** Bimodal   **E.** Normal

1. The heights of men and women in a small village
2. The rate of growth of a child
3. The incidence of heart disease to units of red wine consumption
4. Period of gestation
5. The blood pressures recorded over a year by a GP

3. Consider skewed distributions

a. When the mean is greater than the median the skew is positive
b. When the skew is positive the mean is less than the mode
c. If the skew is negative the mean is greater than the median
d. If the skew is negative the mode is greater than the median

---

GP, general practitioner

EXPLANATION: DISPLAYING DATA

Histograms, scatter plots and pie charts: usually one or more of these methods would be appropriate for displaying information. The one that is chosen should produce the clearest overview, so that the data can be communicated 'at a glance', however it is often just a matter of the preference of the author. As a general rule:

- **Pie charts** are useful for emphasizing how each category compares with the sample as a whole, and can be used for a single series of numbers shown as percentages of the total, the figure opposite shows causes of stroke by subtype
- **Histograms** are good for showing the shape and distribution, as the area under each histogram block is proportional to the number of subjects in that particular group, the figure opposite shows the weights of all staff in a GP practice
- **Scatter plots** can show the association between quantitative variables. If one variable, *a*, is dependent on the other, *b*, then it is usual to plot *a* on the *y* axis and *b* on the *x* axis. The figure opposite of blood urea and creatinine levels in a series of patients suggests that there is a positive association between these two measurements.

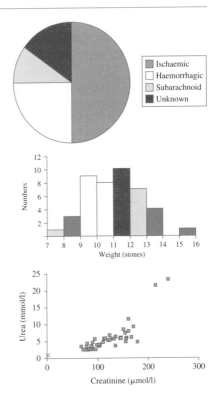

If the majority of results are closer to the top of the range but there are a few spread out at the bottom of the range, it results in a **'negative skew'**. If most of the results are near the bottom of the range the **skew is 'positive'**.

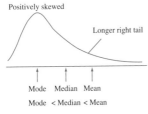

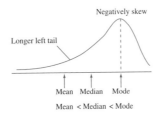

Graphs reproduced with permission from Puri BK, *Statistics for the Health Sciences*, London: WB Saunders, 1996

When data are skewed positively there are a few large numbers or 'outliers' that will affect the calculated average (**mean**). The effect on the mean of a positive skew is to increase it, because the very large numbers are included in the calculation. When ordered according to size, the middle value of the results (**median**) is less affected by a skewed distribution. The number that occurs most (**mode**) is least affected by a skewed distribution (**3**).

Answers

1. 1 – A, 2 – C, 3 – B, 4 – A, 5 – B, 6 – C
2. 1 – D, 2 – B, 3 – A, 4 – C, 5 – E
3. T F F T

4. This is a set of haemoglobin A_{1c} (HbA_{1c}) measurements (in mmol/L) taken at a children's diabetic clinic, used to gauge their blood sugar control over the preceding months. The target HbA_{1c} for this group of children is < 8 mmol/L. The consultant wants to know the extent to which the levels are reaching their target

5.9	15.1	5.9	7.3	6.5	6.2	6.3	6.7
6.9	10.0	5.9	7.1	8.2	5.5	6.6	6.7

a. What is the mean?
b. What is the median?
c. What is the mode?
d. Which of these results gives the best picture of how blood glucose is being controlled in this population of children?

5. The consultant now wants to know what insulin injection devices he should order for his next clinic. He can get individual ones but it would be cheaper to bulk buy the ones he needs the most so he notes down the doses (units) the children are on

16	22	30	30	34	15	30	56
28	30	26	14	18	20	30	30

a. What is the mean?
b. What is the median?
c. What is the mode?
d. Which would be the most useful value for him to know if the pre-filled disposable injections are sold at volumes of 30 units or 78 units?

6. Match the following statements to the most appropriate measure of location

Options

A. Mean   B. Median   C. Mode

1. It takes into account all the data values
2. It is the value that occurs most frequently in a set of data
3. It is used in the calculation of standard deviation
4. There are equal numbers of observations above and below this value
5. It is vulnerable to outliers (values much higher or lower than the average)
6. It is obtained by putting the data in the order from smallest to largest
7. Outliers least affect it
8. It is useful in categorical data to describe the group with the highest frequency

HbA$_{1c}$, Haemoglobin A$_{1c}$

EXPLANATION: CENTRAL LOCATION

In most situations simply listing a series of results does not provide a good quantitative analysis. The **'central location'** of the results can be described better by using the mean, median or mode, depending on which is most suitable.

The **mean** is the calculated average. In a set of data all the values are used to calculate the mean by adding them together and then dividing by the number of data values, sometimes referred to as *n* or the sample size. The mean is represented as $\bar{x}$; and can be calculated using the formula below.

$$\bar{x} = \frac{\text{Sum of individual observations}}{\text{Total number of observations}} = \frac{\Sigma x}{n}$$

In the example given, *n* represents the 16 children who had a blood test at the clinic that morning and the sum of the blood result values is 116.8. The mean is therefore 116.8 divided by 16 which is equal to 7.3 mmol/L **(4a)**.

Advantages of the mean include that it takes into account all of the data and is used as the central point around which the standard deviation is calculated. The main **disadvantage** is that the mean can be greatly affected by outliers, especially in a small sample. In the example most children's HbA_{1c} levels were below the mean but because one child presented that morning with a figure that was high (15.1 mmol/L) the glucose control of the rest of the patients would not be well reflected if the mean value was the only one reported.

The **median** is the measure of the centre of the distribution. To calculate the median the numbers simply need to be put in order and the middle one is chosen. If the number of data values is even the mean of the two middle ones is taken. In the example the numbers 6.6 and 6.7 lie either side of the middle of the data sample so the median is 6.65 mmol/L **(4b)**.

The main **advantage** of the median is that it is more robust to outliers and in small samples like the HbA_{1c} measurements it is much more representative of the glucose control in the group. It is also useful in skewed distributions. However, when the data follow a normal distribution (see page 81) the mean is preferable to the median as a measure of central location.

The **mode** is the value that occurs most frequently. It is very rarely used in statistical analysis of epidemiological data, however the example given shows a useful practical application. The mode is more useful in grouped or categorical data such as age ranges, glove sizes or catheter lengths. It is least affected by outliers, but may not represent values close to the mean or median either.

Answers

4. a – 7.3 mmol/L, b – 6.65 mmol/L, c – 5.9 mmol/L, d – The median
5. a – 27, b – 30, c – 30, d – The mode
6. 1 – A, 2 – C, 3 – A, 4 – B, 5 – A, 6 – B, 7 – C, 8 – C

7. Choose the correct words (i–v) and diagrams (A–E) to match the description of the range of data given (1–5), assuming normal distribution

Options

A.

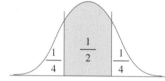

B.

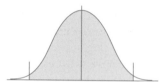

C.

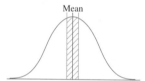

D.

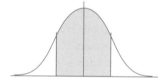

E.

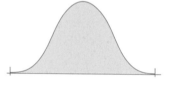

i. Range
ii. Interquartile range
iii. One standard deviation
iv. Two standard deviations
v. Standard error

1. The values that are 34 per cent either side of the mean, representing 68 per cent of the sample population
2. The smallest value to the largest value
3. The value at the top of the first quarter to the bottom of the third quarter when the numbers are put in order from smallest to largest
4. Measures the degree of sampling variability when calculating an estimate of the population mean
5. The values that are 47.5 per cent either side of the mean, representing 95 per cent of the sample population

8. What is the difference between standard deviation and standard error?

SD, standard deviation; SE, standard error; df, degrees of freedom

EXPLANATION: SPREAD

The **range** is the whole dataset from the minimum to the maximum values. It takes into account the outliers and is usually used when representing quantitative data. **Interquartile range** is calculated by putting the data in numerical order and then discarding the lower and upper quarters of the data. The advantage of the interquartile range is that it shows the range of the middle half of the set of measurements, and thus removes the risk of misrepresenting the data distribution due to outliers.

For a continuous measure which follows a normal distribution, the spread is best measured using the **standard deviation** (SD). This measures the average distance that observations are located from the mean and is derived from the variance **(8)**. The **variance** is defined as the sum of the squared differences between the individual measurements and the true mean, divided by the total population size. By subtracting each data point from the mean and then squaring it, the distance from the mean is amplified, while the direction – whether it is smaller or larger than the mean – is removed (squared real numbers are always non-negative). The sample variance is represented by s^2 and is calculated from the data using a similar method as that described above. Instead of dividing by the total population size, s^2 is dividing by the degrees of freedom (df). Because a sample mean has to be calculated in order to estimate a variance or standard deviation, the degrees of freedom are obtained by subtracting 1 from the sample size. The square root of sample variance gives the standard deviation. The data points are expressed as x and Σ is 'sum of'. For further information on notation see the Appendix (page 120).

$$s^2 = \frac{\text{Sum of all squared differences from the mean}}{\text{Sample size} - 1}$$

$$s^2 = \frac{\Sigma(x - \bar{x})^2}{n - 1}$$

The standard deviation is measured in the same units as the mean (e.g. mmHg for blood pressure). When data follow a normal distribution, we would expect that approximately 68 per cent of values will lie within one standard deviation of the mean. Similarly, we would also expect 95 per cent of values will lie within two standard deviations of the mean. To be more exact, 95 per cent of data from a normal distribution lie within plus or minus 1.96 standard deviations of the mean, rather than 2. This is often called the '**normal range**'. **Standard error** (SE) does not measure the degree of spread of a distribution but rather the range of **error** associated with the estimate that is used to describe the data (e.g. standard error of the sample mean) **(8)**. See page 87 for an explanation of standard error. It is included here as it is often mixed up with standard deviation, especially when given in relation to the mean when reporting data in a study.

Answers

7. 1 – Diii, 2 – Ei, 3 – Aii, 4 – Cv, 5 – Biv
8. See explanation

9. For each data group, assign the distribution that best describes the population/
measurements

Options

A. Normal **B.** Binomial **C.** Poisson

1. The weights of all the women in a village
2. The probability of a child in a class having asthma
3. The probability of a child in the school dying from asthma next Tuesday
4. The number of babies born on a particular day who are girls
5. The number of babies conceived this week by all men who had a vasectomy last year
6. Haemoglobin levels in full blood counts of blood donors

10. Using the binomial distribution answer the following questions

In a theoretical situation there are n patients where n is the number of people presenting to the emergency department with right iliac fossa pain (who haven't had a previous appendicectomy) in one week. Each patient has two possible outcomes, appendicectomy or no appendicectomy in the 24 hours after admission. Patients are independent, so the outcome for one patient has no effect on the outcome for another. The probability of having an appendicectomy when presenting with right iliac fossa pain is constant from one patient to another and is 20 per cent or 0.2.

a. In the first week $n = 10$, what is the most likely number that have an appendicectomy?
b. What is the probability that five people had an appendicectomy in that week?
c. What is the probability that eight people had an appendicectomy that week?
d. The following week $n = 20$, what is the probability that 10 had an appendicectomy?
e. What is the probability that eight of those had an appendicectomy?

The hospital changed its policy and the decision was to give antibiotics and delay appendicectomy in non-urgent cases. The probability of having an appendicectomy was then 10 per cent or 0.1. What is the probability that half of the patients had an appendicectomy

f. If $n = 10$? **g.** If $n = 20$?

11. Regarding the Poisson distribution

a. It tends towards the binomial if the probability of an outcome is very large
b. It is most useful for diseases or outcomes that occur commonly
c. It is often used in the study of rare events
d. It is used to describe discrete quantitative data.

EXPLANATION: DISTRIBUTION

Most data on human health and disease are distributed in what is known as the **normal (or Gaussian) distribution**. In a large population the data will appear as the classic 'bell-shaped' curve with a symmetrical distribution, with the majority of values clustered around the mean. Most statistical descriptions of data rely on the assumption that the measurements in the sample conform to the normal distribution. When the numbers are large binomial and Poisson distributions can tend towards the normal distribution.

The **binomial distribution** is a discrete probability distribution and is useful in describing distribution of data where there are two outcomes, such as disease or no disease, death or survival.

The binomial probability for obtaining r successes in N trials is shown below, where $P(r)$ is the probability of exactly r successes, N is the number of events, π is the probability of success on any one trial and ! is factorial[1].

$$P(r) = \frac{N!}{r!(N-r)!}\,\pi^r\,(1-\pi)^{n-r}$$

This formula assumes that the events are dichotomous (fall into only two categories), randomly selected, independent of one another and mutually exclusive (you cannot die and survive!). These outcomes are coded as 1 and 0, respectively. In the following graph the example from question 10 has been used where the probability of appendicectomy was 0.2 and the number of patients 10. For example, the probability of only one of them having an appendectomy equals

$$\frac{10!}{1!(10-1)!}\,0.2^1\,(1-0.2)^{10-1} = 10 \times 0.2 \times (0.8)^9 = 2 \times (0.134) = 0.268$$

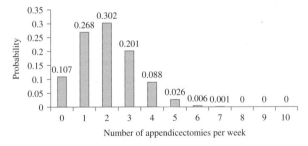

The more patients that present to hospital, the more this distribution tends towards the normal and the less likely it becomes that half of the patients need an appendicectomy.

---

[1]Factorial is the product of all the positive integers less than or equal to n. For example if $n = 4$, $4! = 4 \times 3 \times 2 \times 1$, or 24. When N = 0, 0! = 1.

Continued on page 82

Answers

9. 1 – A, 2 – B, 3 – C, 4 – B, 5 – C, 6 – A
10. a – 2, b – 0.026, c – 0.0001, d – 0.002, e – 0.022, f – 0.0015, g – < 0.0001
11. F F T T

EXPLANATION: DISTRIBUTION Cont'd from page 81

The **Poisson distribution** is useful when the probability of the outcome is very low and/or the population is relatively small. Take the example of men who have had a vasectomy. If 20 000 men have had a vasectomy in the last year, which has a 1 in 2000 failure rate per year, then it is expected that from this population roughly ten babies will be concieved this year. The number of conceptions in any one week is an integer and is therefore usually 0, but in practice may be as many as 3. The mean number of conceptions in a 52-week year is calculated as the sum of the number of weeks multiplied by the number of babies conceived that week, divided by the total number of weeks. For example:

$$= \frac{(44 \times 0) + (5 \times 1) + (2 \times 2) + (1 \times 3)}{52} = \frac{5 + 4 + 3}{52} = 0.23 \text{ conceptions per week}$$

Suppose that before the numbers were counted for the year it was estimated that there was a conception by a man who had had a vasectomy in the previous year roughly once every five weeks. This would estimate the probability of one in a week as 0.2.

Using the formula for the Poisson distribution where μ is the population rate, x is the number of conceptions per week and ! is factorial, a comparison can be made between what was expected and what was observed:

$$P(x) = \frac{\mu^x \times e^{-\mu}}{x!}$$

$P(0) = 0.2^0 \times e^{-0.2} \div 0! = 0.8187$

$P(1) = 0.2^1 \times e^{-0.2} \div 1! = 0.1638$

$P(2) = 0.2^2 \times e^{-0.2} \div 2! = 0.0164$

$P(3) = 0.2^3 \times e^{-0.2} \div 3! = 0.0010$

$P(4) = 0.2^4 \times e^{-0.2} \div 4! = 0.0001$

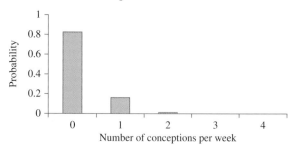

The figure top right shows the Poisson distribution of numbers of conceptions per week, by all men who have had a vasectomy in the last year.

Suppose we increase the population to include all women *and* all men who have been sterilized, by the method of tubal occlusion and vasectomy respectively, in the last year. Tubal occlusion has a failure rate of 1 in 200.

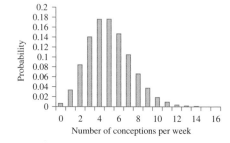

Suppose the estimated risk of conception in any week is now 5 per week. As can be seen by the graph immediately above of the Poisson distribution for $\mu = 5$, the greater the value of μ, the more the distribution tends to the normal or Gaussian distribution.

---

e is a mathematical constant and is the base of natural logarithms. The value of *e* is approximately 2.718 and most calculators have a function for calculating powers of e. For values of *x* that are much smaller than 1.0 but negative, e^{-x} is approximately equal to $1 - x$. If, as in the example above, $x = -0.2$ this approximation is $e^{-0.2} = 1 - 0.2 = 0.8$. Note that this is close to the actual value of 0.8187.

1. Define accuracy

2. Define precision

3. A blood sample was taken from a patient and four different assays were used to measure blood glucose. The true value of the blood glucose was known to be 4.5 mmol/L

   State whether the accuracy and the precision of each assay is high or low

   a. Assay A: 4.6, 4.6, 4.8, 4.5, 4.5, 4.4
   b. Assay B: 4.3, 3.5, 5.3, 4.6, 5.5, 3.7
   c. Assay C: 3.5, 3.6, 3.3, 3.5, 3.4, 3.5
   d. Assay D: 8.5, 6.4, 5.3, 7.6, 4.8, 9.3

4. For the following situations, would it be better to have high accuracy or high precision?

   a. A scientific study investigating the effect of electrolyte concentrations on nerve cell function
   b. A blood pH-measuring assay
   c. An epidemiological study into the relationship between passive smoking and lung cancer

5. Of the following examples, choose the one that gives the most precise information and the one that gives the most accurate information

   a. The weight of newborn babies measured on a recently calibrated weighing machine and recorded to the nearest 0.1 kg
   b. The weight of adults in outpatients weighed using a machine calibrated several years ago but recorded to the nearest gram
   c. Temperatures recorded by a thermometer that always measures 0.8 °C above the patient's actual temperature

EXPLANATION: ACCURACY AND PRECISION AND STATISTICAL SAMPLING

Data can be described in terms of:
- **Accuracy:** how close the measured estimates are to the exact or true value (**1**). For example, when measuring the prevalence of cancer, different studies may produce different values for prevalence. The most accurate studies are those in which the measured value is as close as possible to the true prevalence of cancer
- **Precision:** the reproducibility of a set of measurements (**2**). A precise sample estimate will have a very small random error of estimation. For example, a machine that measures blood glucose levels in blood samples is precise if it will consistently give the same measurement of blood glucose from the same individual's blood sample. However, this machine may not be accurate if it is calibrated such that it always underestimates the value of the blood glucose. Thus a precise but inaccurate method of gathering data will produce a systematic bias in the results.

A dartboard analogy of accuracy and precision is illustrated below.

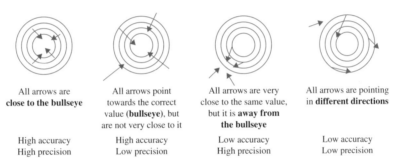

All arrows are **close to the bullseye**	All arrows point towards the correct value (**bullseye**), but are not very close to it	All arrows are very close to the same value, but it is **away from the bullseye**	All arrows are pointing in **different directions**
High accuracy High precision	High accuracy Low precision	Low accuracy High precision	Low accuracy Low precision

Scientific experiments should be highly accurate, in order to obtain true values. Clinical studies often need to be more precise than accurate, as trends and associations are of interest rather than absolute values. Assays and analysers should be highly precise but can be calibrated in order to give accurate readings.

In the case of the blood glucose assay given in question 3 (page 84), the answers to the question are shown in the table opposite (**3**).

	Accuracy	Precision
Assay A	High	High
Assay B	High	Low
Assay C	Low	High
Assay D	Low	Low

Statistical data usually represent a **sample** of a population of interest as it is often impractical or impossible to study the entire population. Through only studying a part of the population, we introduce a **sampling error**. In order to draw valid conclusions it is important to quantify this error. The precision of the sample estimate can be represented by the standard error or confidence intervals.

Answers
1. See explanation
2. See explanation
3. See explanation
4. a – Accuracy, b – Precision, c – Precision
5. a – Most accurate, b – Most precise

6. What is the standard error of the following measures?

    a. Mean cholesterol levels in 40–50 year olds in a GP practice in northern England where:
- Mean = 5.1 mmol/L
- Sample size = 1600
- Standard deviation = 2.3 mmol/L

    b. The proportion of women with skin cancer in women in a small town in Australia where:
- Number of cases of women with skin cancer = 30
- Number of women in study sample = 5700

    c. Mean blood glucose levels on a ward where:
- Mean = 5.1 mmol/L
- Sample size = 16
- Standard deviation = 2.3 mmol/L

    d. Mean peak expiratory flow rates on a respiratory ward where:
- Mean = 400 mL/min
- Sample size = 16
- Standard deviation = 120 mL/min

7. What does a small standard error tell us about the sample estimate of the mean?

    a. That it is highly variable
    b. That it is accurate
    c. That the population standard deviation may be small
    d. That the sample size is probably small
    e. That it is imprecise

8. What will tend to make the standard error larger?

    a. A small variance
    b. A large standard deviation
    c. Imprecise data
    d. Inaccurate data

9. As the size of a random sample increases

    a. The standard deviation decreases
    b. The standard error of the mean decreases
    c. The mean increases
    d. The range may increase
    e. The precision of the parameter estimate increases

GP, general practitioner; SD, standard deviation; SEM, standard error of the mean; SE(p), standard error of the proportion

EXPLANATION: STANDARD ERROR

Example: a study was conducted to investigate the mean systolic blood pressure of a group of hypertensive patients who were treated with a new antihypertensive drug. The study was repeated several times, taking successive samples from the same population treated with the same new drug.

Each sample returned a slightly different value for the mean systolic blood pressure: these values are estimates of the true mean of the blood pressure in the whole population and can be displayed as a histogram, as shown opposite.

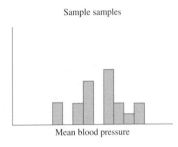

If the distribution of blood pressure in the population follows a normal distribution, the estimates of the means from each sample should also follow a normal distributions known as the **sampling distribution of the mean**. If the overall sample size is very large, it will follow a normal distribution, regardless of the distribution of the original data in the population.

The variability of this distribution is known as the **standard error of the mean** (SEM). As it is not usually practical to repeat studies many times to obtain estimates of the mean from a number of different samples, the SEM can be estimated using the standard deviation (SD).

$$SEM = SD/\sqrt{n}$$

where n is the sample size.

From this calculation it is evident that the standard error becomes smaller when the variability of the data (SD) remains constant and the sample size increases.

The smaller the standard error, the more **precise** is the sample estimate. This is in contrast to the SD which represents the variability of the primary observations. The standard error **does not** reflect the **accuracy** of the data.

If a study investigating the proportion of individuals with a given characteristic is repeated several times using different samples from the same population, the estimates of the true proportion will approximate a normal distribution, known as the **sampling distribution of a proportion**. The estimates have a variability that is represented by the **standard error of the proportion** (SE(p)). This value can be approximated from a single sample using the following equation:

$$SE(p) = \sqrt{(p(1 - p)/n)}$$

Answers

6. a – SEM = 2.3/√1600 = 0.0575 mmol/L; b – Proportion, p = 30/5700 = 0.0053; SE(p) = √(0.0053 × (1 − 0.0053)/5700) = 0.00096 women; c – SEM = 2.3/√16 = 0.58 mmol/L; d – SEM = 120/√16 = 30 mL/min

7. F F T F F

8. F T T F

9. F T F T T

10. Using the normal distribution provided in the Appendix (page 124), calculate the confidence intervals for the following datasets

    a. The 95 per cent confidence interval (CI) for the forced expiratory volume (FEV_1) of children with asthma, where the mean is 1.47 L, the standard deviation is 0.34 L and the sample size is 1089

    b. The 99 per cent CI for the proportion of babies born with birth defects to mothers who had an infection during pregnancy, where the number of babies with birth defects is 7 and the total number of babies in the study is 43. (NB: In the normal distribution, 99 per cent of the data lie within 2.58 standard deviations of the mean.)

11. Using the t-distribution provided in the Appendix (page 125), calculate the CI for the length of time to recovery to full fitness: a study of 10 athletes with sports injuries, mean length of time of recovery to full fitness of 36 days, standard deviation of 21.4 days

12. Interpret the following results

A study was conducted to investigate whether there was a difference in mean systolic blood pressure between a group of army recruits who smoke and a group who do not smoke. The means in two groups were adjusted for age and other risk factors for hypertension.

Smoking status	Mean systolic blood pressure (mmHg)	Standard deviation	Sample size
Yes	149	17	70
No	131	10	70

    a. What is the standard error of each of the two means?
    b. What are the 95 per cent CIs for the two means?
    c. What can you conclude from these CIs?

13. A 95 per cent CI for a mean

    A. Is narrower than a 99 per cent CI
    B. Is a useful way of describing the precision of a study
    C. Includes 95 per cent of the observations in a study
    D. Will include the population mean 95 per cent of the time in repeated samples

14. Several different studies investigated the effect of a new statin drug on cholesterol levels in samples of patients with similar characteristics. Choose the set of results that shows the most convincing reduction in cholesterol level

    A. 2 mmol/L 95 per cent CI 1.1 to 2.2   D. 5 mmol/L 99 per cent CI of 0.5 to 3.1
    B. 2 mmol/L 99 per cent CI 1.1 to 2.2   E. 5 mmol/L 95 per cent CI of 4.6 to 5.3
    C. 5 mmol/L 95 per cent CI −0.1 to 9.5

CI, confidence interval; FEV_1, forced expiratory volume; SE, standard error; SEM, standard error of the mean; SD, standard deviation

EXPLANATION: CONFIDENCE INTERVALS

A **confidence interval** (CI) represents both the precision and the accuracy of an estimate. It is derived from the standard error but is expressed in such a way to help us to picture the sampling variation in the estimate more easily. The **interval** represents the range of values within which we can be confident that the true value of our population parameter lies. The **confidence** with which, to a certain degree, we can believe in this interval is specified by a percentage representing the probability that the CI contains the true population parameter.

The degree of confidence often used is 95 per cent. Here there is a 95 per cent chance that the theoretical interval contains the true population parameter. It is often claimed that one can be 95 per cent certain that the true population parameter lies within the 95 per cent CI obtained from a single sample. This is not, however, strictly correct. As the population parameter is a fixed unknown quantity, it either lies inside or outside the 95 per cent CI. If 100 independent random samples were drawn from the same population, we would expect 95 of these to include the true population parameter. It is also possible to obtain intervals using other degrees of confidence. For example, 99 per cent CIs would make a more certain statement about the likely magnitude of the true population parameter.

$$\text{95 per cent CI for the mean} = \bar{x} - (1.96 \times \text{SEM}), \bar{x} + (1.96 \times \text{SEM})$$

The CI for the example given in question **10a** (page 88) is calculated as follows:

$$1.47 \pm (1.96 \times 0.34/\sqrt{1089}) = 1.47 \pm 0.020$$

where mean = 1.47 L, SD = 0.34 L, sample size is 1089, and so SEM = $0.34/\sqrt{1089}$.

The 95 per cent CI is 1.45 to 1.49 L.

The CI for the example given in question **10b** (page 88) is calculated as follows:

Proportion p = 7/43 = 0.163, SE of p = $\sqrt{[0.163 \times (1 - 0.163)/43]}$ = 0.056

Lower limit of 99% CI is 0.163 − (2.58 × 0.056) = 0.019, upper limit of 99% CI is 0.163 + (2.58 × 0.056) = 0.307

The 99 per cent CI for the proprotion of babies born with birth defects is 0.019 to 0.307 or 1.9% to 30.7%

When the sample size is large, the sampling distribution of the mean approximates the normal distribution. In the normal distribution, 95 per cent of values lie within plus or minus 1.96 standard deviations of the mean. The CI is calculated from the equation below, where SEM is the standard error of the mean and the multiplier, 1.96, is the percentile of the normal distribution that gives a 95 per cent CI.

Continued on page 90

Answers

10. See explanation   **11.** See explanation (page 90)
12. a – Smokers: SE = $17/\sqrt{70}$ = 2.0; non-smokers: SE = $10/\sqrt{70}$ = 1.2, b – Smokers: 95 per cent CI = 149 ± (1.96 × 2.0) = 149 ± 3.92. 95 per cent CI is 145 to 153; non-smokers: 95 per cent CI = 131 ± (1.96 × 1.2) = 131 ± 2.35. 95 per cent CI is 129 to 133, c – The SEM is smaller for non-smokers than for smokers, suggesting that the estimate of the mean blood pressure is more precise for non-smokers than smokers. The narrower CI for non-smokers suggests that the estimate is also more accurate than for smokers
13. F T F T   **14.** E

EXPLANATION: CONFIDENCE INTERVALS Cont'd from page 90

When the sample size is small (e.g. less than 20), the data may not be so normally distributed, and the variance of the population may not be known. Therefore a different probability curve, the **Student's t-distribution** is used. The t-distribution is similar to the normal distribution, but is more spread out with longer tails. The multiplier, $t_{0.05}$, is the percentile of the t-distribution that gives a two-tailed probability of 0.05.

$$\text{95 per cent CI for the mean} = \bar{x} - (t_{0.05} \times \text{SEM}),\ \bar{x} + (t_{0.05} \times \text{SEM})$$

To calculate 99 per cent CIs, one would multiply the SEM by a t-value corresponding to a two-tailed probability of 0.01.

The t-distribution can be used to calculate CIs **(11)** for mean length of time to recovery to full fitness. For a t-distribution with $n-1$ degrees of freedom ($10 - 1 = 9$), $t_{0.05} = 2.26$:

$$\text{95 per cent CI for the mean} = 36 \pm 2.26 \times (21.4/\sqrt{10}) = 36 \pm 15.3 \text{ days}$$

95 per cent CI is 20.7 to 51.3 days.

As for the mean, the sampling distribution of the proportion approximates the normal distribution when the sample size is large. Therefore the **95 per cent CI for the proportion** is given by:

$$p - [1.96 \times \sqrt{(p(1-p)/n)}],\ p + [1.96 \times \sqrt{(p(1-p)/n)}])$$

where n is the sample size.

If the sample size is small, the binomial distribution is used to calculate exact CIs for proportions.

The width of the CI represents the **precision** of the sample estimate:
• Wide CI: imprecise estimate
• Narrow CI: precise estimate.

As the width of the CI is derived from the standard error, increasing the sample size or decreasing the variability of the original data will decrease the width of the CI, reflecting the increased precision of the estimate. The higher the degree of confidence, such as a 99 per cent CI, the stronger our belief that the true parameter lies between the interval values given.

CI, confidence interval; SEM, standard error of the mean

HYPOTHESIS TESTING

SECTION 11 HYPOTHESIS TESTING

1. Define null hypothesis and alternative hypothesis

2. Put the stages of doing a hypothesis test into the correct order

    A. Interpret the *P*-value
    B. Calculate the test statistic
    C. Define the null and alternative hypotheses
    D. Collect the relevant data
    E. Obtain the *P*-value from the appropriate probability distribution curve

3. Comparing hypothesis tests and confidence intervals

    A. Hypothesis tests are easier to calculate
    B. A hypothesis test can give an exact value for the *P*-value
    C. A confidence interval does not tell you about the significance of the results
    D. A hypothesis test gives an idea of the precision of the results whereas the confidence interval cannot
    E. A hypothesis test gives you an idea of the likely magnitude of a population parameter whereas a confidence interval cannot

4. What is the difference between a one-tailed test and a two-tailed test?

5. What are the advantages of a two-tailed test?

6. Why would one use a one-tailed test?

H_0, null hypothesis; H_1, alternative hypothesis; intelligence CI, confidence interval

EXPLANATION: PRINCIPLES OF HYPOTHESIS TESTING

The purpose of an epidemiological study is often to investigate the relationship between a variable of interest and an outcome of interest. The investigator usually begins the study with an idea or a theory as to the possible nature of the relationship. This theory can be approached by **hypothesis testing**.

A statistical method, known as a **hypothesis test**, is used to quantify the strength of evidence against the null hypothesis, based on the data that have been collected in the study. The hypothesis test involves comparing the mean sample estimate, $\bar{x}$, with a hypothetical value of a true population parameter.

Stages of hypothesis testing are as follows (2):
1. Define the null and alternative hypotheses (H_0 and H_1 respectively)
2. Collect relevant data
3. Calculate the test statistic specific for the null hypothesis
4. Compare the value of the test statistic to values from a known probability distribution to obtain a *P*-value
5. Interpret the *P*-value and the results.

Definitions are as follows:
- **Null hypothesis, H_0:** a statement about the true population parameter of interest, for example the true mean, μ (1). The null hypothesis might state that there is no difference in the true means of two populations: $\mu_1 = \mu_0$
- **Alternative hypothesis, H_1:** any hypothesis that differs from H_0, for example the true population means are different: $\mu_1 \neq \mu_0$ (1)
- **Two-tailed test:** the direction of the relationship stated by the alternative hypothesis is not specified (4). This is normally preferred as it is often difficult to predict the direction of a true association in advance of the study, as by definition statistical studies involve a degree of uncertainty. A two-tailed test therefore has stronger statistical credentials (5)
- **One-tailed test:** the direction of the relationship is specified by the altenative hypothesis (4). A one-tailed test is used occasionally when the results can only occur in one direction. An example might be when testing a new drug treatment for a condition in which the only outcome without treatment is death, i.e. the drug can have either no effect or can increase survival (6).

A **hypothesis test** provides an exact value of the *P*-value and therefore the exact degree of certainty we can hold in our results, i.e. the accuracy of the results. The **95 per cent CI** specifies the range over which we can be 95 per cent certain that the true population parameter lies relative to our estimate of the population parameter. This is equivalent to the certainty provided by a *P*-value < 0.05, but also indicates the degree of precision of the estimate. CIs tell us about the likely magnitude of the estimated parameter, whereas hypothesis tests do not.

Answers

1. See explanation	**4.** See explanation
2. C D B E A	**5.** See explanation
3. F T F F F	**6.** See explanation

7. Match the study questions (1–5) to the most appropriate statistical test

Options

A. ANOVA
B. Chi-squared test for 3×2 table
C. 2-sample unpaired z-test
D. 2-sample paired z-test
E. Chi-squared test for 2×2 table

1. A new drug for lowering mean blood pressure is being compared with a placebo in a crossover trial
2. Is there a higher risk of breast cancer in women who take the pill versus women who do not?
3. Is the proportion of smokers different in France, Britain and Germany?
4. Is the mean BMI of 15-year-olds in Scotland greater than the mean BMI of 15-year-olds in England?
5. Three different drugs for the treatment of hypercholesteraemia are being compared using mean cholesterol levels across the groups

8. Calculate the test statistic for the following data

An unmatched study into a new lipid-lowering drug (use the data in the table below)
- H_0: triglyceride levels are the same in the population of individuals receiving lipid-lowering treatment as in the population who are not receiving treatment
- H_1: triglyceride levels are different in the treated population versus the untreated population

	Mean serum triglyceride (mmol/L)	Standard deviation (mmol/L)	Sample size
Treated	4.6	1.5	54
Untreated	5.4	1.5	67

ANOVA, analysis of variance; SD, standard deviation; H_0, null hypothesis; H_1, alternative hypothesis; BMI, body mass index

INTERPRETATION OF DATA

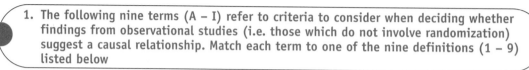

SECTION 12 — INTERPRETATION OF DATA

1. The following nine terms (A – I) refer to criteria to consider when deciding whether findings from observational studies (i.e. those which do not involve randomization) suggest a causal relationship. Match each term to one of the nine definitions (1 – 9) listed below

Options

A. Temporality
B. Strength of association
C. Dose–response
D. Plausibility
E. Consistency
F. Specificity
G. Coherence
H. Experiment
I. Analogy

1. The relationship can be modified by experimental interference
2. Agrees with prior strong evidence of a similar association
3. The risk factor must precede disease
4. A single exposure or risk factor has a specific effect
5. Consistent with current understanding of biological or pathological processes
6. Increased exposure to risk factor increases the risk of disease
7. The results are replicable or in accordance with those of other, similar studies
8. Large relative risk or correlation coefficient, with small standard error
9. Agrees with existing knowledge and widely accepted theories

2. Of the following, choose which values give a measure of the strength of an association

a. Odds ratio
b. Relative risk
c. Standard deviation
d. Confidence interval
e. Correlation coefficient

EXPLANATION: RISK

Risk is the probability of an outcome, usually a harmful one, over a fixed period of time. It is calculated from the results of a cohort study as the number of events during the defined study period divided by the number of individuals at risk of that event.

Absolute risk = number developing disease in study period/total number in cohort. For example, the absolute risk of a 50-year-old man having a myocardial infarction (MI) in 1 year is the number of men aged 50 years having an MI in 1 year divided by the number of men in the whole population who are 50 years old.

Relative risk = absolute risk in group 1/absolute risk in group 2. The relative risk compares the risk in two groups. One is referred to as the 'exposed' group and the other, usually the initial or control group, is the 'unexposed' group. For example, if the absolute risk of an MI within 1 year for men aged 50 is 0.01 per cent and the absolute risk for men aged 60 is 0.02 per cent, the relative risk for men aged 60 compared to men aged 50 would be 0.02/0.01 = 2.00.

Relative risk reduction = absolute risk reduction/absolute risk in group 1. When a 'new' treatment is introduced, a trial is often carried out to compare it to the 'gold standard', namely the 'old' treatment that is currently most widely accepted as being the best. The objective is to calculate the relative risk of disease in those taking the 'old' treatment compared to that in the 'new' treatment group. The relative risk reduction is the proportion of the risk with the 'old' treatment that has been eliminated by using the 'new' treatment. For example, if the risk of an MI in a population taking 'old' treatment for hypertension is 0.05 per cent and the 'new' treatment brings the risk down to 0.03 per cent, the relative risk reduction is (0.05 − 0.03)/0.05 × 100 or 40 per cent.

Absolute risk reduction = absolute risk in group 1 − absolute risk in group 2. The absolute risk reduction can sometimes give a more realistic indication of the effect of a new treatment than the relative risk reduction. Using the same example above, any person who is told they could reduce their risk by 40 per cent would probably take the 'new' treatment. However, if the reduction in risk is converted to absolute risk reduction this equals 0.02 per cent (0.05 − 0.03). Such a small reduction in absolute risk may appear less favourable to an individual in the light of the cost or any additional side-effects of the 'new' drug.

Numbers needed to treat (NNT) = 1/absolute risk reduction. When presenting a choice of treatment options to a patient there may be cases when neither the relative risk reduction nor the absolute risk reduction gives them a good idea as to what it means to them as an individual. Sometimes by putting it into the 'user friendly' context of numbers needed to treat, the difference between old and new treatments can be understood more readily. Using the example above, NNT = 1/0.02 = 50, therefore the doctor can tell the patient that if he or she gives 50 people the new medication for 1 year he or she will prevent 1 myocardial infarction (MI).

Answers

9. D is ten times as effective as the other options as they all convert to a number needed to treat of 170

10. a − 0.6 per cent, b − ((60 − 54)/60) × 100) = 10 per cent, c − 0.06 per cent, d − 1/0.0006 = 1667 people, e − Probably the relative risk reduction (10 per cent)

11. a − Absolute risk group B = 10/80 = 12.5 per cent; absolute risk group A = 5/50 = 10 per cent; absolute risk reduction = 12.5 − 10 = 2.5 per cent, b − Relative risk reduction = absolute risk reduction/absolute risk group B = 2.5/12.5 = 0.2 or 20 per cent, c − NNT = 40

12. For what type of data is correlation a useful measure of association?

13. What would the correlation coefficient, r, be for the following theoretical linear relationships?

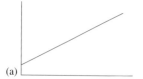
(a)

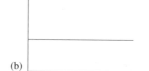
(b)

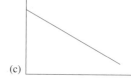
(c)

14. What do these values of r imply about the relationships displayed in graphs (a), (b) and (c)?

15. What is the equation for a linear relationship between two variables, x and y?

16. A study into the effects of a new drug on serum cholesterol was conducted on 20 subjects and the following results obtained:

Regression line: $y = 0.7 - 0.6x$; standard error of the slope = 0.28
Answer the following questions:

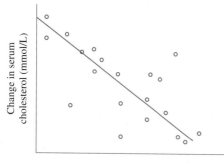

Drug dose (mg)

a. Define the null and alternative hypotheses for this study

b. Does this drug have a significant effect on serum cholesterol level at the 5 per cent level? Would you accept or reject the null hypothesis?

c. What would be the expected change in serum cholesterol if the following doses of the new drug were given to the patient: 1 mg, 2 mg, 5 mg, 10 mg?

d. How could you explain the increase in serum cholesterol at low drug doses?

EXPLANATION: CORRELATION AND LINEAR REGRESSION

Correlation measures strength of linear association between two numerical variables. If two variables have a **linear** relationship the data points will form a straight line when plotted on Cartesian axes **(12)**. Degree of correlation can be calculated using the **Pearson correlation coefficient, r,** which can have a value between +1 and −1, where +1 = positive correlation (risk increases linearly with increasing exposure), or −1 = negative correlation (risk decreases linearly with increasing exposure); $r = 0$ represents absence of any linear correlation. This is illustrated below.

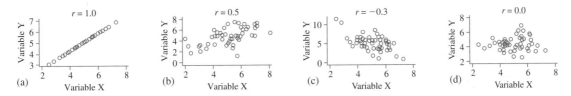

Graphs reproduced with kind permission from Everitt BS and Palmer CR (eds), *Encyclopaedic Companion to Medical Statistics*, Great Britain: Hodder Education, 2005

The square of the correlation coefficient, r^2, represents how much of the variability in y can be accounted for by variability in x, in other words, how well the data fit the line. For example, a study shows that there is a positive association between the number of cigarettes smoked and systolic blood pressure with correlation coefficient $r = + 0.5$. Therefore $r^2 = 0.25$, suggesting that 25 per cent of the increase in blood pressure can be accounted for by the increased number of cigarettes smoked. It is very important to remember that two variables having a high correlation coefficient does not mean that one causes the other.

When one of the variables is considered to be dependent on the other, the relationship can be analysed using **linear regression**. This is the process of attempting to fit a straight line to the observed data points, such that the data can be represented by the equation

$$y = bx + a \quad \textbf{(15)}$$

where x is the independent variable whose value can be measured accurately, y is the dependent variable, b is the slope of the line and a is the intercept on the y axis when $x = 0$.

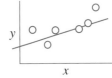

Linear regression analysis is often achieved by finding the **best fit**: the straight line that minimizes the **sum of the squares** of the vertical deviations of each data point from the line. These deviations are known as the **residuals** and they are squared so as to avoid any cancellations between data points that are above and below the line. The resulting regression equation is valid for values of y and x that are within the observed range of data. Extrapolating to predict values of y from values of x beyond the data range can lead to inappropriate and incorrect answers.

Answers

12. See explanation **13.** a − Positive, $r = +1$, b − zero $r = 0$, c − Negative $r = −1$ **14.** a − Positively correlated, b − No correlation, c − Negatively correlated **15.** See explanation

16. a − Null hypothesis: drug has no effect on serum cholesterol; alternative hypothesis: drug dose influences serum cholesterol, b − Test statistic = 0.6/0.28 = 2.14, df = 20 − 2 = 18, $P < 0.05$, i.e. results are significant at the 5 per cent level: reject the null hypothesis, c − An increase of 0.1 mmol/L, a decrease of 0.5 mmol/L, a decrease of 2.3 mmol/L, a decrease of 5.3 mmol/L, d − With no drug treatment, ($x = 0$), cholesterol levels can be expected to rise by 0.7 mmol/L. Very low drug doses are insufficient to coonteract this rise.

17. Assuming a correlation exists in the following examples, which examples are appropriate for testing correlation by linear regression (true or false)

   a. The correlation between resting heart rate and square root of the number of miles cycled by different cyclists on a weekly basis, assuming the relationship is linear and there are no confounding variables

   b. The relationship between blood pressure and blood cholesterol levels of the people who went to their GP last week; some people presented as many as three times

   c. The relationship between height, and a rare disease, y, that does affect stature but is not found to be normally distributed in the population

   d. The relationship between blood levels of 'liver markers' and liver damage; where liver markers rise exponentially with increasing liver damage

18. For the examples a–d in question 17 give the main reason, if there is one, using the list of assumptions below (1–4), why it is not appropriate to use linear regression analysis

   1. The relationship must be linear

   2. Observations must be independent, there cannot be different numbers of observations made on the same individuals

   3. Other, confounding variables, must be excluded

   4. The y values are normally distributed in the population

19. Are the following true or false?

   a. Predictions can be derived from information that is correlated linearly

   b. If you know x and the equation for the relationship you can calculate y

   c. If you know y and the equation you cannot calculate x

   d. The results can be 'extrapolated' or extended to predict values for x and y outside the original range

df, degrees of freedom; SE, standard error; GP, general practitioner

SUMMARY OF STATISTICAL TESTS

QUANTITATIVE DATA

Test	Circumstances	Assumptions	Null hypothesis	Test statistic
One-sample z-test (or t-test if small sample)	One group of numerical data. 'Is the mean different from expected?'	Normal distribution; reasonable sample size	Sample mean ($\bar{x}$) = hypothesized value for mean (μ)	$z = \dfrac{(\bar{x} - \mu)}{s/\sqrt{n}}$ n = sample size, s = estimated standard deviation
Two-sample paired z-test (or t-test if small sample)	Two groups of paired numerical data. 'Is there a difference in means between the pairs?'	Normal distribution; reasonable sample size; the two groups are the same size	Mean of differences between sample pairs = zero	$z = \dfrac{\bar{d}}{s/\sqrt{n}}$ n = number of paired differences, $\bar{d}$ = mean difference in pairs, s = estimated standard deviation of paired differences
Two-sample unpaired z-test (or t-test if small sample)	Two groups of unpaired numerical data. 'Is there a difference between the means of the two groups?'	Normal distribution of data in both groups; groups have same variance; reasonable sample sizes	Difference between sample means = zero	$z = \dfrac{\bar{x}_1 - \bar{x}_2}{\sqrt{(SE_1{}^2 + SE_2{}^2)}}$
ANOVA (analysis of variance)	Multiple groups of numerical data: single test. 'Is there a difference between the means in each group?'	Mean is same in each group		F distribution: a complex calculation which can be carried out using computer packages.

CATEGORICAL DATA

Test	Circumstances	Assumptions	Null hypothesis	Notation
One-sample z-test	Two categories, one group of data 'Is there a difference in the proportion of the sample with the characteristic of interest compared to a hypothesized value for the proportion?'	Data follow the binomial distribution which approximates the normal distribution if the sample size is large enough	Population proportion, π = hypothesized proportion, π_1	$$z = \frac{|p - \pi| - (1/2n)}{\sqrt{(p(1-p)/n)}}$$ p = population with characteristic of interest = r/n; r = number with characteristic, n = sample size
Two-sample chi-squared test χ^2	Two categories with > 2 groups of data. (See table on page 123)	Groups are independent and mutually exclusive; the expected frequency in each category > 5	There is no difference between the observed frequency and the expected frequency (frequency expected if there was no difference between the two groups)	$$\chi^2 = \frac{\Sigma(|O - E| - 1/2)^2}{E}$$ df = $n - 1$ O = observed frequency, E = expected frequency
	> 2 categories; data expressed in an $r \times c$ table	Mutually exclusive categories; expected frequency > 5 in 80 per cent of the categories		$$\chi^2 = \frac{\Sigma(|O - E|)^2}{E}$$ df = $(r - 1) \times (c - 1)$ when using chi-squared test df should be given
McNemar's test	Two categories; two groups of data; categories not mutually exclusive (paired)			
Fisher's exact test	Two categories; 2+ groups of data; expected frequency < 5	Mutually exclusive categories		

df, degrees of freedom

CHI-SQUARED CONTINGENCY TABLE

	Group 1	Group 2	Total
Characteristic present (observed frequency, O)	a	b	$a + b$
Characteristic absent	c	d	$c + d$
Total	$a + c$	$b + d$	$a + b + c + d$
Proportion with characteristic	$p_1 = a/(a + c)$	$p_2 = b/(b + d)$	$p = a + b/(a + b + c + d)$
Expected frequency (E)	$E_1 = (a + c) \times p$	$E_2 = (b + d) \times p$	

STATISTICAL TABLES

THE STANDARD NORMAL DISTRIBUTION

z	Two-tailed *P*-value 0.00	0.01	0.02	0.03	0.04	0.05	0.06	0.07	0.08	0.09
0.0	1.0000	0.9920	0.9840	0.9761	0.9681	0.9601	0.9522	0.9442	0.9362	0.9283
0.1	0.9203	0.9124	0.9045	0.8966	0.8887	0.8808	0.8729	0.8650	0.8572	0.8493
0.2	0.8415	0.8337	0.8259	0.8181	0.8103	0.8026	0.7949	0.7872	0.7795	0.7718
0.3	0.7642	0.7566	0.7490	0.7414	0.7339	0.7263	0.7188	0.7114	0.7039	0.6965
0.4	0.6892	0.6818	0.6745	0.6672	0.6599	0.6527	0.6455	0.6384	0.6312	0.6241
0.5	0.6171	0.6101	0.6031	0.5961	0.5892	0.5823	0.5755	0.5687	0.5619	0.5552
0.6	0.5485	0.5419	0.5353	0.5287	0.5222	0.5157	0.5093	0.5029	0.4965	0.4902
0.7	0.4839	0.4777	0.4715	0.4654	0.4593	0.4533	0.4473	0.4413	0.4354	0.4295
0.8	0.4237	0.4179	0.4122	0.4065	0.4009	0.3953	0.3898	0.3843	0.3789	0.3735
0.9	0.3681	0.3628	0.3576	0.3524	0.3472	0.3421	0.3371	0.3320	0.3271	0.3222
1.0	0.3173	0.3125	0.3077	0.3030	0.2983	0.2937	0.2891	0.2846	0.2801	0.2757
1.1	0.2713	0.2670	0.2627	0.2585	0.2543	0.2501	0.2460	0.2420	0.2380	0.2340
1.2	0.2301	0.2263	0.2225	0.2187	0.2150	0.2113	0.2077	0.2041	0.2005	0.1971
1.3	0.1936	0.1902	0.1868	0.1835	0.1802	0.1770	0.1738	0.1707	0.1676	0.1645
1.4	0.1615	0.1585	0.1556	0.1527	0.1499	0.1471	0.1443	0.1416	0.1389	0.1362
1.5	0.1336	0.1310	0.1285	0.1260	0.1236	0.1211	0.1188	0.1164	0.1141	0.1118
1.6	0.1096	0.1074	0.1052	0.1031	0.1010	0.0989	0.0969	0.0949	0.0930	0.0910
1.7	0.0891	0.0873	0.0854	0.0836	0.0819	0.0801	0.0784	0.0767	0.0751	0.0735
1.8	0.0719	0.0703	0.0688	0.0672	0.0658	0.0643	0.0629	0.0615	0.0601	0.0588
1.9	0.0574	0.0561	0.0549	0.0536	0.0524	0.0512	0.0500	0.0488	0.0477	0.0466
2.0	0.0455	0.0444	0.0434	0.0424	0.0414	0.0404	0.0394	0.0385	0.0375	0.0366
2.1	0.0357	0.0349	0.0340	0.0332	0.0324	0.0316	0.0308	0.0300	0.0293	0.0285
2.2	0.0278	0.0271	0.0264	0.0257	0.0251	0.0244	0.0238	0.0232	0.0226	0.0220
2.3	0.0214	0.0209	0.0203	0.0198	0.0193	0.0188	0.0183	0.0178	0.0173	0.0168
2.4	0.0164	0.0160	0.0155	0.0151	0.0147	0.0143	0.0139	0.0135	0.0131	0.0128
2.5	0.0124	0.0121	0.0117	0.0114	0.0111	0.0108	0.0105	0.0102	0.0099	0.0096
2.6	0.0093	0.0091	0.0088	0.0085	0.0083	0.0080	0.0078	0.0076	0.0074	0.0071
2.7	0.0069	0.0067	0.0065	0.0063	0.0061	0.0060	0.0058	0.0056	0.0054	0.0053
2.8	0.0051	0.0050	0.0048	0.0047	0.0045	0.0044	0.0042	0.0041	0.0040	0.0039
2.9	0.0037	0.0036	0.0035	0.0034	0.0033	0.0032	0.0031	0.0030	0.0029	0.0028
3.0	0.0027	0.0026	0.0025	0.0024	0.0024	0.0023	0.0022	0.0021	0.0021	0.0020

df, degrees of freedom

STUDENT'S *t*-DISTRIBUTION

df	Two-tailed *P*-value 0.1	0.05	0.01	0.001
1	6.31	12.71	63.66	636.58
2	2.92	4.30	9.92	31.60
3	2.35	3.18	5.84	12.92
4	2.13	2.78	4.60	8.61
5	2.02	2.57	4.03	6.87
6	1.94	2.45	3.71	5.96
7	1.89	2.36	3.50	5.41
8	1.86	2.31	3.36	5.04
9	1.83	2.26	3.25	4.78
10	1.81	2.23	3.17	4.59
11	1.80	2.20	3.11	4.44
12	1.78	2.18	3.05	4.32
13	1.77	2.16	3.01	4.22
14	1.76	2.14	2.98	4.14
15	1.75	2.13	2.95	4.07
16	1.75	2.12	2.92	4.01
17	1.74	2.11	2.90	3.97
18	1.73	2.10	2.88	3.92
19	1.73	2.09	2.86	3.88
20	1.72	2.09	2.85	3.85
21	1.72	2.08	2.83	3.82
22	1.72	2.07	2.82	3.79
23	1.71	2.07	2.81	3.77
24	1.71	2.06	2.80	3.75
25	1.71	2.06	2.79	3.73
26	1.71	2.06	2.78	3.71
27	1.70	2.05	2.77	3.69
28	1.70	2.05	2.76	3.67
29	1.70	2.05	2.76	3.66
30	1.70	2.04	2.75	3.65
40	1.68	2.02	2.70	3.55
50	1.68	2.01	2.68	3.50
100	1.66	1.98	2.63	3.39
1000	1.65	1.96	2.58	3.30

df, degrees of freedom

THE CHI-SQUARED DISTRIBUTION

df	Two-tailed P-value			
	0.1	0.05	0.01	0.001
1	2.71	3.84	6.63	10.83
2	4.61	5.99	9.21	13.82
3	6.25	7.81	11.34	16.27
4	7.78	9.49	13.28	18.47
5	9.24	11.07	15.09	20.51
6	10.64	12.59	16.81	22.46
7	12.02	14.07	18.48	24.32
8	13.36	15.51	20.09	26.12
9	14.68	16.92	21.67	27.88
10	15.99	18.31	23.21	29.59
11	17.28	19.68	24.73	31.26
12	18.55	21.03	26.22	32.91
13	19.81	22.36	27.69	34.53
14	21.06	23.68	29.14	36.12
15	22.31	25.00	30.58	37.70
16	23.54	26.30	32.00	39.25
17	24.77	27.59	33.41	40.79
18	25.99	28.87	34.81	42.31
19	27.20	30.14	36.19	43.82
20	28.41	31.41	37.57	45.31
21	29.62	32.67	38.93	46.80
22	30.81	33.92	40.29	48.27
23	32.01	35.17	41.64	49.73
24	33.20	36.42	42.98	51.18
25	34.38	37.65	44.31	52.62
26	35.56	38.89	45.64	54.05
27	36.74	40.11	46.96	55.48
28	37.92	41.34	48.28	56.89
29	39.09	42.56	49.59	58.30
30	40.26	43.77	50.89	59.70

df, degrees of freedom

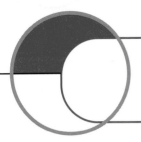

INDEX